Health Services in
the United States

Health Services in the United States

REVISED
AND ENLARGED
FIRST EDITION

Florence A. Wilson
Duncan Neuhauser

Ballinger Publishing Company • Cambridge, Massachusetts
A Subsidiary of J.B. Lippincott Company

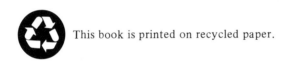
Copyright © 1976 by Ballinger Publishing Company. All rights reserved. No part of this publication may be reproduced, stored in a retrieval system, or transmitted in any form or by any means, electronic mechanical photocopy, recording or otherwise, without the prior written consent of the publisher.

International Standard Book Number: 0-88410-700-0

Library of Congress Catalog Card Number: 76-42472

Printed in the United States of America

Library of Congress Cataloging in Publication Data

Wilson, Florence A
  Health services in the United States.

  Includes bibliographical references and index.
  1. Medical care—United States. I. Neuhauser, Duncan, joint author. II. Title.
RA395.A3W54 1976   362.1'0973   76-42472
ISBN 0-88410-700-0

Contents

List of Figures

List of Diagrams

List of Tables

Preface

This description of health services in the United States was originally developed for graduate students at the Harvard School of Public Health. It attempts to provide a concise summary of major components of health care in this country. Much of this information has only been available in widely scattered, often elusive documents, or exists as common knowledge among health professionals who learned it by experience or word of mouth.

One might refer to this document as the anatomy of American health services. It stops short of being physiology, that is, how the system works. It stops short of being pathology, that is, how and where the services fail to work. Finally, it does not include the techniques which managers, professionals, or consumers might use to operate, modify or change health services.

We have attempted to be as objective and dispassionate as possible. However, this is often exceedingly difficult. One can scarcely write a word in this field without it being the potential source of controversy and debate. For example, take the title of this document. We might have referred to the "U.S. Health Services System," but there is an argument as to whether it is a "system" or a "non-system." The social scientists refer to it as a "system," implying that it has a boundary, component parts, and relationships. The reformers refer to it as a "non-system" implying that it is chaotic and in need of a reorganization along more rational lines.* We have tried to avoid

*We might have used health services industry instead of system, but one ideological implication of the word "industry" is that health services are just like the automobile or steel industry and they are or should be all under the control of the market place.

taking sides but since much of the content has been the focus of political or ideological debates the task is difficult.

A document such as this has other inherent problems. For example, much effort has gone into making it as brief as possible, which leads to the dilemma of what to include and what to exclude and where to place the emphasis. Here our general rule has been to focus on those areas which are most important to the understanding of current issues. Some readers therefore may feel that their own occupation or organization has not been covered to the depth they would like. Also, since one of the distinguishing characteristics of American health services is their great diversity and variety, many general descriptive statements may be to some degree misleading or wrong; yet, if every exception were cited this document would be unduly long. Finally, some of the material will soon be affected by ongoing changes in laws and institutions. Despite these problems, we hope this endeavor will prove useful.

Comments, criticisms and suggestions concerning this initial endeavor will be welcomed, and may be communicated directly to the authors. The first two chapters, most of the third, and the eighth were done by D.N. The remaining chapters, and section on nurses, are by F.W.

Finally, we wish to express our appreciation to the Ford Foundation Urban Studies Seminar for assistance in the development of this book.

Harvard School of Public Health   Duncan Neuhauser, Ph.D.
Boston   Florence A. Wilson, M.D.

Health Services in
the United States

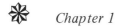 *Chapter 1*

Health Care Institutions

1. INTRODUCTION

American health services can be viewed as an interdependent subcomponent of the larger social system of the United States. As such, health services interfaces with other subcomponents including:

Education. Schools, Colleges and Universities educate health workers and define their roles and conduct health-related research.

Economic. Technology, the labor market, and the mix of independent for-profit and not-for-profit corporations. Transportation, Capital Markets.

Law. Common law and legislated law.

Government. Transfer payments such as Medicare and Medicaid programs. Delivery Systems at the Federal, State and Local level.

Population. Numbers, age, sex and racial distribution, urbanization, birth, death rates, morbidity and mortality.

Environment. Natural resources, climate, pollution, distance between providers and patients.

Culture. History, values, religion, and attitudes about health care and health related behavior, such as smoking, alcohol consumption, and exercise.

This chapter describes health care institutions, like hospitals and nursing homes. Chapter Two describes health care professions and occupations. Chapter Three describes the ways that health care is paid for. The remaining chapters are concerned with the federal, state and local government, with ambulatory care, voluntary agencies, quality and cost control, and the pharmaceutical and supply industry.

2. TYPES OF HEALTH CARE INSTITUTIONS
(Organizations, Facilities)

There is a wide variety of health facilities which vary according to the type of patient served and services provided.

Inpatient and Residential Facilities

- Hospitals, general and special
- Nursing Care and Related Homes
  Nursing care home, personal care home with nursing, domiciliary care home, personal care home without nursing
- Other Inpatient Health Facilities
  Facility for Alcoholics
  Facility for Blind and/or Deaf
  Facility for Dependent Children
  Facility for Drug Abusers
  Facility for the Emotionally Disturbed
  Facility for the Mentally Retarded
  Facility for the Physically Handicapped
  Facility for Unwed Mothers
  Juvenile Correctional Facility
  Orphanage

Other Facilities and Services (Non-Institutional and Ambulatory Care—See Chapter 6)

Ambulance Services
Blood Banks

Clinical (Medical) Laboratories
Comprehensive Health Services Programs
   Community Mental Health Center
   Migrant Health Program
   Neighborhood Health Center
Dental Group Practice
Dental Laboratories
Family Planning Facilities
Home Health Services (Home Health Agency)
   Including, home care programs, home health aide service, community nursing service, visiting nurse association
Hospital Outpatient Services
   Ancillary Department
   Emergency Department
   Outpatient Department (Ambulatory Care Department)
Medical Group Practices
Opticianry Establishments
Pharmacies (See Chapter 9)
Poison Control Centers
Psychiatric Outpatient Services (Hospital Affiliated or Free-Standing)
Rehabilitation Facilities including Sheltered Workshop and Speech and Hearing Center
Suicide Prevention Centers including Crisis Intervention Agency, Suicide Hotline and Suicide Prevention Program
Pharmaceutical Manufacturers and Distributors (See Chapter 9)
Hospital Supply Industry (See Chapter 9)
Insurance and Prepayment Organization (See Chapter 3)

Source: *Health Resources Statistics, 1974.* National Center for Health Statistics, U.S. Department of HEW, PHS, HSMHA (Rockville, Maryland), 1974, pp. 528–533.

General Hospitals and General Nursing Care Institution

The following two definitions are used by the American Hospital Association.[1] Other definitions exist. Drawing the line between different types of facilities is somewhat arbitrary because the boundary lines are not completely clear.

[1] American Hospital Association, *Classification of Health Care Institutions*, Chicago, 1974 edition.

General Hospitals

Definition. An establishment that provides—through an organized medical staff, permanent facilities that include inpatient beds, medical services, and continuous nursing services—diagnosis and treatment, both surgical and nonsurgical, for patients who have any of a variety of medical conditions.

Essential Characteristics for Classification

1. The primary function of the institution is to provide diagnosis and treatment, both surgical and nonsurgical, for patients who have any of a variety of medical conditions.
2. Inpatient beds are maintained in the institution.
3. There is a governing authority legally responsible for the conduct of the institution.
4. There is an administrator to whom the governing authority delegates the full-time responsibility for the operation of the institution in accordance with established policy.
5. There is an organized medical staff to which the governing authority delegates responsibility for maintaining proper standards of medical care.
6. Each patient is admitted on the medical authority of, and his care is under the direction of, a member of the medical staff.
7. The nursing services are under the direction of a full-time registered professional nurse.
8. Registered professional nurse supervision and other nursing services are continuous.
9. A medical record is maintained for each patient.
10. Pharmacy services are maintained in or by the institution and supervised by a licensed pharmicist.
11. Diagnostic x-ray services, with facilities and staff able to conduct a variety of procedures, are maintained in the institution.
12. Clinical laboratory services, with facilities and staff able to conduct a variety of tests and procedures, are maintained in or by the institution, and anatomical pathology services are regularly and conveniently available.
13. Operating room services, with facilities and staff, are maintained in the institution.
14. Food served to patients meet their nutritional requirements, and modified diets are regularly available.

General Nursing Care Institution

Definition. An establishment that provides—through an organized medical staff, a medical director, or a medical adviser and permanent facilities that include inpatient beds, medical services, continuous nursing services, and health-related services—diagnosis and treatment for patients who are not in an acute phase of illness but who primarily require skilled nursing care on an inpatient basis.

Essential Characteristics for Classification

1. The primary function of the institution is to provide treatment for patients who are not in an acute phase of illness but who primarily require skilled nursing care on an inpatient basis.
2. The institution maintains inpatient beds.
3. There is a governing authority legally responsible for the conduct of the institution.
4. There is an administrator to whom the governing authority delegates the full-time responsibility for the operation of the institution in accordance with established policy.
5. There is an organized medical staff, or one that serves the institution through an affiliation, or a medical director, to which the governing authority delegates responsibility for maintaining proper standards of medical care; or there is a medical adviser.
6. Each patient is admitted on the medical authority of, and his care is under the direction of, a physician.
7. The nursing services are under the direction of a full-time registered professional nurse.
8. There is registered professional nurse supervision on a daily basis. Licensed graduate nurse supervision and other nursing services are continuous.
9. A medical record is maintained for each patient.
10. There are arrangements for providing necessary rehabilitative services.
11. There are arrangements for providing health-related services.
12. There are arrangements for obtaining necessary clinical laboratory and diagnostic x-ray services.
13. There is control of the storage, dispensing, and administration of all medications.
14. Food served to patients meets their nutritional requirements, and modified diets are regularly available.

3. TYPES OF HOSPITALS

Hospitals can be characterized in a number of different ways, including:*

1. Ownership
2. Type of Patient Treated and Services Provided
3. Average Length of Patient Stay
4. Medical and Osteopathic
5. Teaching and Non-Teaching

The American Hospital system provides an incredibly wide variety of types of hospitals; the most important in terms of volume of patients cared for are the state long-term mental hospitals and the voluntary short-term general community hospitals.

Because there are so many variations according to types of ownership, organization, and types of patient treated, there are numerous exceptions to what follows.

Hospital Ownership

Federal

Department of Defense (DOD): Army, Navy, Air Force. The Department of Defense operates hospitals and clinics whose primary purpose is to provide care for active and retired members of the seven uniformed services: Army, Navy, Marine Corps, Air Force, Coast Guard, Commissioned Corps of the National Oceanic and Atmosphere Administration and the Commissioned Corps of the Public Health Service and their dependents. 9.9 million people were eligible for free care in 1972 under these programs, including 2.5 million active duty members, 1.0 million retired members, 3.5 dependents of active duty, and 2.2 dependents of the retired and 0.7 million survivors of uniform services members. The CHAMPUS program provides funding for dependents and retired members to receive care in private hospitals.

The Army, Navy and Air Force have their own hospital and health

*The National Center for Health Statistics defines a hospital as:

A hospital is defined as a facility with at least six beds that is licensed by the State as a hospital or that is operated as a hospital by a Federal or State agency and is therefore not subject to State or local licensing laws.

Health Resources Statistics, 1974, p. 340.

Government Ownership

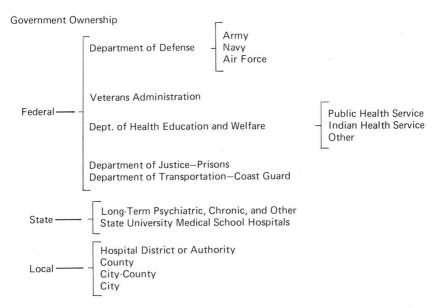

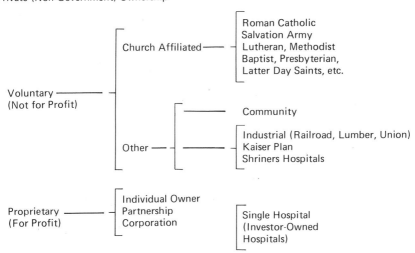

Figure 1-1. Hospitals by Type of Ownership

Source: James A. Hamilton, *Patterns of Hospital Ownership and Control*, (Minneapolis: University of Minnesota Press, 1961).

care systems with small clinics and inpatient services on military bases, hospitals serving larger areas, and large medical centers serving regions.

Veteran's Administration (VA). Provides a system of health care for veterans including 169 hospitals (136 general hospitals, 33 psychiatric hospitals, 61,378 medical and surgical beds, 36,122 psychiatric beds in 1973). Inpatient care was provided to 980,000 patients in 1973. In addition, there are 76 nursing homes and 16 domiciliary homes, with 7,000 beds and 12,000 beds respectively in 1973. There has been a major increase in the use of outpatient facilities. The VA serves an eligible population of 29 million veterans. Veterans with service-connected injuries and those aged 65 or more have the highest priority for VA care. Veterans with non-service connected disabilities may be treated in VA facilities if they attest that they are unable to pay for hospitalization. Veterans aged 65 or over may use Medicare benefits in private hospitals or use a VA hospital, regardless of ability to pay.

The VA also has about 200 clinics. It has facilities in all fifty states. Over 150,000 personnel are employed in the VA system. There are major teaching programs for physicians and allied health personnel. VA medical research activities are particularly noteworthy. VA institutions are affiliated with over 80 medical schools and about half the 5,000 full-time VA doctors hold academic appointments in medical schools.

The following types of patients are eligible for care in VA hospitals, which are scattered throughout the U.S.:

1. Those requiring treatment for military service-connected disabilities.
2. Those requiring treatment for non-service-connected conditions who were either discharged from military service for a disability incurred or aggravated in the line of duty, or who have a compensable service-connected disability
3. Other veterans with wartime service who require treatment for non-service-connected conditions, if they are not able to pay for private hospital care. They must indicate on an affidavit that they are unable to pay for hospital care and include a statement of their assets.
4. Military personnel transferred from military hospitals to continue treatment, who are in the process of being discharged from the armed forces

About 70 percent of VA patients are below the poverty level.

Department of Health, Education and Welfare

- *Patient Care and Special Health Services* program funded through Health Services Administration, operates 8 *Public Health Service Hospitals*, 30 clinics and 98 health units (1974). These facilities provide care for American merchant seamen, personnel of the Coast Guard and the Public Health Service Commissioned Corps. This program also operates a long-term care leprosarium in Louisiana.
- *The Indian Health Service* provides care for about 480 thousand American Indians and Alaska natives. It operates 51 hospitals and 83 health centers.
- *The Alcohol, Drug Abuse and Mental Health Administration* cares for neuropsychiatric patients at the Clinical Research Center, Lexington, Kentucky.

Department of Justice. The Federal Bureau of Prisons provides medical services for prisoners in federal institutions, including the 1,000 bed referral Medical Center for Federal Prisoners.

Other. St. Elizabeths Hospital (Washington, D.C.) a psychiatric hospital for District of Columbia and Virgin Island residents. (HEW)

The Coast Guard (Department of Transportation) operates its own hospitals and clinics in addition to using PHS and military hospitals.*

Admissions to Federal inpatient facilities, 1974, under major Federal programs are as follows:

Department of HEW	
Patient Care and Special Health Services	22,888
Indian Health Service	74,600
Alcohol, Drug Abuse and Mental Health	1,268
Department of Defense	1,035,260
Department of Justice	7,490
Veterans Administration	1,050,243

*Louise B. Russell, *et al. Federal Health Spending 1969-1974.* Center for Health Policy Studies, National Planning Association, Washington, D.C., 1974.

State

Long Term. Every state operates one or more state hospitals emphasizing institutional care of the mentally ill, the retarded, and tuberculosis patients. They are run by departments, boards, or administrative agencies of state governments, such as departments of health or welfare. There are also state schools for the blind, deaf, and mentally deficient, and infirmaries or hospitals connected with state reformatories and prisons. Residents of the state for a certain period of time who are unable to pay for care on a private basis are eligible. Admission to mental hospitals can be a voluntary decision on the part of the patient, or, more frequently, an involuntary commitment by a court on the recommendation of a court-appointed board of examiners, which considers petitions from the patient's family and testimony of psychiatrists in a commitment hearing.

Short Term. Primarily acute care general hospitals controlled by state medical schools as a primary source of patients for educating students, such as the University Hospital in Ann Arbor, Michigan, of the University of Michigan Medical School.

Local

District. These are similar to school, sanitary, water, etc., districts. They are political subdivisions set up for the purpose of maintaining a hospital with the power to tax the population in the district. They are governed by a board of directors which is elected by district residents. As such, they are independent of city, county, or state government. This is not a common form of organization except in a few states, e.g., California.

County. These hospitals are run by the county board of supervisors. They include the large urban hospitals for the indigent, like Cook County Hospital in Chicago. They also include many smaller, rural hospitals which care for both private patients and indigent patients.

City-County. Controlled jointly by municipal and county governments, often for indigent patients.

City. Owned by municipal government and managed by an appointed board of citizens. They include hospitals primarily for the indigent and hospitals for both indigent and paying patients.

Voluntary ("Voluntary" and "nonprofit" are usually used interchangeably.)

Church. A number of religious groups own, operate, or own and operate hospitals. The Roman Catholic Church is foremost of these groups in terms of number of hospitals.

Roman Catholic hospitals are owned and operated by over 100 different sisterhoods (religious orders, or communities of women bound together within the Church by vows of poverty, chastity, and obedience). Most religious orders are expected to be self-sufficient and are relatively independent of each other; however, all orders must abide by the canon laws of the Church. The Mother Superior (sometimes Mother General or Mother Provincial) of the order is usually president of the hospital governing board. A sister usually administers the hospital (although this is changing) and sisters work in a variety of capacities within the hospital, although they are usually only a small fraction of the hospital's total work force. (There are brotherhoods which run hospitals as well, e.g., The Alexian Brothers.) Some Roman Catholic hospitals are owned and managed by a Diocese or Archdiocese (the regional organization of the Church).

Other Religious Groups. Over a dozen different Protestant denominations own, operate, or own and operate hospitals. Jewish hospitals are not owned or controlled by religious organizations. Instead, they are independent community hospitals supported by the Jewish community.

Community Hospitals. These are independent, nonprofit hospital corporations or associations composed of public-spirited citizens who are interested in providing hospital care for their community and who organized solely for that purpose. These hospitals, governed by nonprofit associations or corporations which are usually open to any interested citizen, require a small yearly contribution, and can have up to several thousand members, usually meet once a year for the purpose of electing new members of the hospital board of trustees or directors. The board typically has 5 to 15 members, meets monthly, has by-laws, and elects its own officers. The board is subdivided into various committees: executive, finance, fund-raising, etc. The executive committee typically meets weekly, appoints the administrator, and approves the appointments of physicians to the hospital medical staff. The administrator, in turn, appoints department heads and is in charge of the day-to-day operation of the hospital. There are perhaps as many variations on this theme as there are community hospitals.

Other. A number of hospitals are run by industrial corporations for their employees (railroads, logging) and by unions for their members. The Shriners (the Ancient Arabic Order of Nobles of the Mystic Shrine of North America) own and operate a number of hospitals for crippled children under the age of 14 who are unable to pay their full costs and who have a possibility of cure or rehabilitation to self-sufficiency.

Cooperative Hospitals. These are controlled by the users of health services, and provide comprehensive care, require prepayment by members, and utilize group medical practice. These include the Group Health Association of Washington, D.C., the Group Health Cooperative of Puget Sound, and the Kaiser Foundation.

Proprietary (synonymous with for-profit). Hospitals have traditionally been owned by one physician (*individual owner*) or a group of physicians (as a *partnership* or *corporation*), who usually use these hospitals for the care of their own patients.[2]

A new development in the last decade has been the growth of *investor-owned hospital corporations*, which are sometimes called *hospital chains*. The stock of these corporations is publicly bought and sold on stock exchanges. They may own and manage hospitals, nursing homes, health maintenance organizations, clinical laboratories, and such, in the United States and abroad. Some of their recent growth has been in the area of *management contracts*, where they contractually undertake to manage a hospital which they do not own. These corporations have central offices and specialized staff. They publicly emphasize their managerial expertise.

Hospitals by Type of Patient Treated

- General Medical and Surgical (General Hospitals)
- Hospital Unit of an Institution (Prison Hospital, College Infirmary)
- Psychiatric
- Tuberculosis
- Narcotic Addiction, Addictive Diseases
- Geriatric
- Maternity

[2] B. Steinwald and D. Neuhauser. "The Role of the Proprietary Hospital." *Journal of Law and Contemporary Problems*, August, 1970. Also, Clark V. Havighurst (Editor) *Health Care.* New York: Oceana Publications, 1972.

- Eye, Ear, Nose and Throat
- Physical Rehabilitation
- Orthopedic
- Chronic and Convalescent
- Institutions for Mental Retardation
- Epilepsy
- Alcoholism
- Other
- Children's Hospitals, including: General; Unit of an Institution; Psychiatric; Tuberculosis; Eye, Ear, Nose and Throat; Physical Rehabilitation; Orthopedic; Chronic and Convalescent; Other.

Osteopathic Hospitals. (See section on Osteopathy). Osteopathic hospitals are those staffed by Doctors of Osteopathy and are either of the nonprofit community or proprietary types. They are mostly general hospitals.

Patient Payment Status and Types of Accommodation

Patient Status[3] Based on Ability to Pay

- *Self-Pay* patients pay their own hospital bill without recourse to insurance benefits.
- *Third Party Paid* patients have part or all of their care paid for by insurance. (Third party to the patient and the practitioner).
- *Medically Indigent* patients are those who have enough income to live on but are unable to meet the costs of medical care.
- *Indigent Patients* do not have enough money to live on. Indigent patients are sometimes called poor patients, charity patients, service patients, or ward patients.

Types of Accommodation—*Private, Semi-Private,* and *Ward Patients.* This distinction refers to the type of room the patient occupies in the hospital.

- A *private patient* occupies a room by himself.
- A *semi-private patient* usually occupies a room with one to three other people (or beds).
- A *ward patient* occupies a room with three or more other people (or beds). *Private* and *ward* also refer to different physician-patient arrangements. Private patients have their own doctor who they pay for services rendered. Ward (or service or charity) patients are

[3] The words "case" and "patient" are used synonymously.

cared for by the doctors in charge of the unit, often including interns and residents, and are supervised by staff physicians.[4]

Teaching Hospitals. Although definitions vary, teaching hospital usually refers to the existence of an approved physician *internship* and/or *residency* program in the hospital. It can also refer to the clinical teaching of medical students in the hospital (medical school affiliation). Medical school affiliation may be by agreement or by ownership, the medical school owning and operating the hospital (for example, the University of Chicago clinics). Hospitals may also be involved in teaching student nurses and other types of personnel. *House staff* refers to both interns and residents combined, as distinct from the *full-time staff* who spend their full working time in the hospital and often may be paid by the hospital or medical school (again, definitions vary), and as distinct from the visiting staff, who are in private practice earning their livelihood through charges to patients.

Frequently Used Hospital Statistics.[5]   *Patient Days (Patient Bed Days).* The total number of inpatient days of care given in a specified time period. For example, if there were 50 patients in the hospital for each day for 10 days this would be 500 patient days for this time period.

Hospital Beds. The average number of beds, cribs, and pediatric bassinets (excluding bassinets for newborn babies) regularly maintained (set up and staffed for use) for inpatients during a period of time (usually a year).

Bassinets. Bassinets, incubators, and isolators for newborn babies in a nursery.

Admissions. Number of patients accepted for inpatient service in a period of time (excluding births).

Discharges and Deaths. Number of inpatients leaving the hospital in a period of time. This usually excludes newborn babies.

Census (Average Daily Census). Number of inpatients receiving care on an average day (excluding newborns). This is usually calculated by counting the number of patients in the hospital every midnight (*midnight census*).

---

[4] See American Association of Medical Record Librarians, *Glossary of Hospital Terms*, (Chicago: The Association, 1969).

[5] American Hospital Association, The Guide Issue, *JAHA*, yearly.

Occupancy. The ratio of census to beds, usually as a percentage of beds in use.

Average Length of Stay (ALOS). Average stay, in days, of inpatients in a given time period. This can be calculated by dividing the number of patient days by either the number of admissions or the number of discharges and deaths.

Available Bed Days. The average number of beds available for use times the number of days in a given time period. Thus, a 100-bed hospital would have 36,500 available bed days per year.

Staffing Ratio. The total number of hospital employees (full-time equivalents) divided by the average daily census.

Per Diem Cost, Cost Per Patient Day. The cost of running the hospital divided by the number of patient days in that time period. Various adjustments or corrections in the cost figures are sometimes made in order to compare hospitals.

Inpatients and Outpatients. Outpatients can also be called *ambulatory* patients or *clinic* patients. Sometimes clinic patients refers to medically indigent patients who use the clinics and associated inpatient ward services. In other hospitals the clinics may be open to both paying and indigent ambulatory patients.

Waiting List. An ordered list of patients awaiting admission to the hospital. The number of patients on that list.

Some Other Definitions

Short-Term and Long-Term Hospitals. These differ according to the average length of stay of the inpatients. According to the American Hospital Association's definition, in short-term hospitals over 50 percent of all patients admitted stay less than 30 days.

Hospital Service Charge (Per Diem Charge). The basic price per day for inpatient care, usually including food, basic nursing care, administrative overhead, use of the facility: those services used by all patients. *Ancillary Charges* are for special diagnostic and treatment services, such as lab tests, X-rays, operating room, etc.

The medical staff in all but the smallest hospitals is divided by specialty, for example surgery medicine, obstetrics gynecology, psychiatry, general practice etc.[6] Each of these services or departments has a chief of services and a more or less formally structured

---

[6] For specialties see the section on *Physicians* under *Health Manpower*

organization with meetings, responsibilities, and policies. These specialty groupings may be associated with separate groups of inpatient beds reserved for the appropriate patients. For example, beds will be set aside solely for the use of obstetrical patients and this unit will be associated with the obstetrical department of the medical staff. Other specialties may or may not have beds especially designated for their patients. If not their patients would be mixed together with those under the care of other specialists.

4. HOSPITALS: INTERNAL ORGANIZATION

The General Hospital: Its Internal Characteristics

The Medical Staff. The medical staff consists primarily of physicians and may include dentists, psychologists, podiatrists, etc. For a doctor to be *on the staff* of a hospital, he must have *hospital privileges* or *hospital admitting privileges.*

An *open staff* is one where any licensed physician may admit his private patient to the hospital and care for him there. Although this used to be widespread, it is now very rare.

A *closed staff* means that only those physicians whose applications for staff membership have been reviewed and approved by the hospital's governing body (board of trustees) may admit and care for patients. This is now the customary arrangement.

Usually a physician who desires to be on the staff of the hospital makes out a written application. This application is reviewed by a credentials' committee of the medical staff, which checks to see if he is duly licensed to practice medicine. This committee of staff doctors makes an advisory recommendation to the board of trustees, which has the final legal authority to specify staff membership.[7]

Many hospitals have a number of different classifications of medical staff, which can include the following:

- *active staff*—the regular membership
- *associate*—junior membership
- *consulting*—doctor can consult but not admit
- *courtesy*—for a doctor who only occasionally uses the hospital

[7] Again, it is important to remember that there are endless variations on these ways of doing things. What follows can be viewed as typical arrangements.

- *emeritus*—for doctors retired from the active staff
- *house staff*—interns and residents
- *honorary*—for noted doctors not heavily involved in the hospital

Usually staff appointments are renewable yearly. In exchange for the privilege of admitting patients to the hospital, staff physicians are usually asked to give some of their time in service to the hospital, often in the form of committee membership, chief of services, teaching, research, etc. The amount of this service varies substantially with the hospital.

The *Medical Staff By-Laws* are rules and regulations which govern the behavior of physicians on the hospital's staff. These by-laws are approved by the governing body of the hospital, with the advice of the medical staff. These by-laws vary from hospital to hospital, but they generally include the following:

1. *Statement of Purpose:* To insure quality of care, to maintain staff self-government and educational standards.
2. *Statement Concerning Membership:* Qualifications, ethical conduct, terms of appointment, procedure for appointment and termination, appeal procedure.
3. *Descriptive Outline of the Medical Staff Organization:* Categories of membership, listing and description of clinical departments.
4. *Statement Concerning Medical Staff Functions:* To be accomplished through medical staff committees which are likely to include (a) executive, (b) credentials, (c) joint conference, (d) accreditation, (e) medical records, tissue, and audit reviews, (f) utilization, (g) infections, (h) pharmacy, (i) other.
5. *Statement of Delineation of Privileges:* Saying what range of patients and treatments each physician may care for and use.
6. *Statement about Staff Meetings:* Including (a) annual meeting, (b) regular departmental, (c) special, (d) attendance records, (e) rules of order, and (f) agenda.
7. *Rules and Regulations:* For (a) keeping accurate and complete medical records, (b) insuring that tissue removed by operation is sent to the laboratory, (c) insuring routine physical examination of all patients on admission and the recording of a pre-operative diagnosis before surgery, (d) insuring that surgical patients give consent to the operation, (e) insuring consultations on special cases, and (f) insuring that physician orders are written and signed.

The staff usually has an overall president and/or chief of staff. The staff is usually subdivided by department (medicine, surgery, pediatrics, obstetrics, gynecology, etc.), each with a chief of service. There may also be a director of medical education.

These positions may be appointed by the governing body or elected by the medical staff or some combination. They may be salaried in full, in part, or not at all. They may have an office in the hospital or may not.

Medical Staff Committees. Some Important Examples include: *Executive Committee* consists of the chiefs of service, elected members of the staff, and other officers, and is the senior decision-making body of the medical staff.

Joint Conference Committee includes officers of the medical staff and members of the governing board for the purpose of maintaining communications between board and staff. Not all hospitals have this committee.

Credentials Committee reviews applications for staff membership.

Utilization Review Committee reviews patient records to insure that it is necessary for patients to be in the hospital. Having such a committee is a requirement for participation in Medicare.

Tissue Committee reviews surgical specimens to see if the tissue was diseased or not. It is presumed to be a check on surgical performance.

Medical Records, Infection, and Pharmacy Committees review performance in these areas of the hospital in connection with medical staff activities.

The extent of committees, full-time chiefs of staff, and formalized medical staff rules depends on the size of the hospital. Larger hospitals tend to be more structured and formalized.

The Medical Record. The medical record is the written record of the patient's progress. Each patient seen in a hospital and in a doctor's private office has a record. When the patient is in the hospital, this record is kept at the nursing station and is also referred to as the *patient's chart.* When the patient is not in the hospital, the chart becomes the medical record and is stored in the Medical Records Department.

The medical record usually includes several separate sections; among them are the following:

- *admissions form*—patient's name, age, sex, address, attending physician, admission diagnosis, etc.
- *past history*—relevant family, mental, and personal history; previous illnesses and hospitalizations; allergies

- *system history*—previous problems associated with different parts of the body
- *physical examination*—present condition of different parts of the body
- *summary sheet*—chief complaint, present illness, significant findings, diagnostic impression, and suggested program
- *daily record of temperature, pulse and respiration (TPR)*—weight, food, treatment, and medication
- *laboratory data*—laboratory test results
- *treatment record*—doctor's orders, and his required signature; description of operation and other procedures
- *nurse's notes*—observations of patient's behavior and condition
- *discharge note*—disposition (i.e., next steps in treatment), discharge summary of hospitalization, discharge diagnosis, and physician's signature
- *other special reports*—e.g., autopsy report

The Problem-Oriented Medical Record, recently developed by Dr. Lawrence L. Weed,[8] is a reorganization of the contents of the medical record. It changes the focus from the admitting diagnosis to a numbered list of all the patient's problems (active and inactive). By so doing, it attempts to avoid guessing at initial diagnoses. Progress toward the resolution of each of these problems is pursued as the focus of the patient's record. Dr. Weed argues that this form of record is better for teaching students and compels attention to the full range of the patient's problems.

Miscellaneous Hospital Terminology

Emergency Admission, emergency surgery must be cared for immediately, in contrast to an *elective admission* (elective surgery) which may be delayed without harm to the patient.

Rounds. "To make rounds" constitutes a physician's visit to the bedsides of his hospitalized patients to note their progress.

Ward Rounds, Teaching Rounds. The teaching physician's bedside review of patients for the purpose of supervising and instructing house staff and medical students (*bedside teaching*).

Grand Rounds. In a hospital, the (usually) weekly description, review, and discussion of a patient (*presentation of a case*), in an auditorium, to all the medical staff of the hospital for the purpose of education.

[8] Lawrence L. Weed, M.D., Medical Records, *Medical Education and Patient Care*, (The Press of Case Western Reserve University; distributed by Year Book Medical Publishers, Chicago, Illinois).

Clinico-Pathological Conference (CPC). The physical examination and diagnostic test results are described before the full medical staff; an expert then analyzes these findings and attempts a diagnosis. Then the pathologist reports his diagnosis, based on tissue examination.

A *referral* is when one doctor sends a patient to another doctor who specializes in the appropriate area. In doing so, the referring doctor hands over primary responsibility for the patient to that specialist. A *consultation* consists of seeking advice from a specialist (a consultant) without relinquishing primary responsibility for the patient.

Fee splitting is a practice widely condemned as unethical. It refers to the consultant's returning a part of his fee to the referring physician as a reward for making the referral.

References

"Hospital Accreditation References," 1964 edition, American Hospital Association, Chicago, Illinois, 1964.

"General Principles of Medical Staff Organization," American Medical Association, Chicago, Illinois, December 1964.

C. Wesley Eisele (editor), *The Medical Staff in the Modern Hospital*, (New York: McGraw-Hill, 1967).

"Model Medical Staff By-Laws, Rules and Regulations," Joint Commission on Accreditation of Hospitals, Chicago, Illinois, 1964.

Milton Roemer and Jay W. Friedman, *Doctors in Hospitals*, (Baltimore, Md.: The Johns Hopkins Press, 1971).

T.R. Ponton, *The Medical Staff in the Hospital*, (Chicago, Illinois: The Physicians Record Company, 1953).

5. HOSPITAL DEPARTMENTS AND SERVICES

Hospitals are often organized in two different ways simultaneously. The first way the hospital is organized is that patients are grouped together by specialty in wards, floors or nursing units. For example the hospitals' patients and doctors may be grouped into medical, surgical, pediatric and other specialties. In addition to these inpatient groupings there are groupings of ambulatory patients which may include an emergency unit and various outpatient clinics.

Secondly hospital personnel are grouped into departments such as

Table 1-1. An Example of an Organization Chart for a Large Community General Hospital*

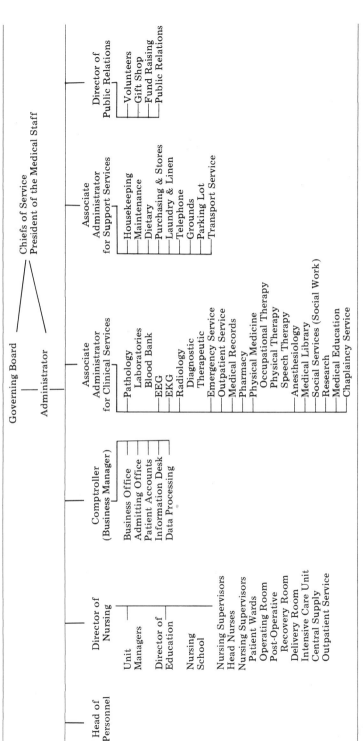

*The internal organization of the medical staff is not shown.
Other hospital services could include: Abortion Services, Burn Care Unit, Cobalt Therapy, Dental Services, Extended Care Unit, Family Planning Service, Genetic Counseling, Home Care Program, Hospital Auxiliary, Inhalation Therapy, Intensive Cardiac Care Unit, Open-Heart Surgery Facilities, Organ Bank, Podiatrist Services, Premature Nursery, Psychiatric Services, Psychiatric Foster and/or Home Care, Radio-isotope Facility (Diagnostic, Therapeutic), Radium Therapy, Rehabilitation Services, Renal Dialysis, Self-Care Unit.

nursing, dietary, laboratory etc. These departments provide services to all patients who need them. The section that follows will primarily focus on this second way in which hospitals are organized.

This distinction becomes confusing for such units as radiology, laboratories, anesthesiology, physical medicine etc. which include both specialized physicians and other hospital personnel.

The words *department* and *services* are used differently in different hospitals.

Sometimes *services* refers to separate groupings of patients, some personnel, and doctors: for example, surgical, medical, obstetrical, emergency, private, or outpatient services. Most other groupings of hospital personnel would be called *departments*, for example, the X-ray, nursing, and dietary departments.

Sometimes *services* is defined to include personnel who provide services directly to patients: for example, the nursing and dietary services. Sometimes they are all referred to as *departments*: for example, the surgical department. Sometimes several departments or services are administratively grouped together to form *divisions*.

Excluding medical staff, the departments of the hospital can be grouped under Nursing Services, Ancillary Services, Administration and Support Services.[9] The overall, day-to-day responsibility for the performance of these services lies with the administrator, his associates, and assistants who, in turn, answer to the hospital's governing board. The administrator also may be called *matron* (archaic), *superintendent* (now rare), *general director*, or *president*. Some hospitals have a president, who is concerned with long-term planning, community relations, board of trustees relationships, etc., and an executive vice president, who is responsible for the day-to-day internal management of the hospital. One example of the organization of a large community general hospital is shown in Table 1-1. There are probably as many variations in organization as there are hospitals, with respect to which services are offered, how they are grouped, and where they are located within the hospital.

Nursing Services (Department of Nursing, Division of Nursing)

The *Nursing Department* is the single largest component of the hospital. It includes a *director of nursing*, responsible for the whole

---

[9] For descriptions of types of personnel and their education, see the section on "Health Manpower."

department; *nursing supervisors*, responsible for several nursing units, each of which is run by a *head nurse*; other nursing personnel on the *nursing unit* (*patient floor* and *ward* are sometimes used to refer to groups of patient rooms in the same place).

Nursing units are often divided up by medical specialty, often including medical, surgical, obstetrical, pediatric, and psychiatric units. There may also be separate units for infectious diseases, *intensive care units* (ICU), and *coronary care units* (CCU). The head nurse directs a group of nursing personnel, including professional nurses (RNs), practical nurses (LPNs), nursing aides, and male orderlies. There is usually a *ward clerk* who copes with the paperwork at the nursing station, where the medical records and medications are kept. There also may be student nurses gaining practical experience and a *unit manager* who carries out a variety of managerial activities, thereby freeing nursing personnel for the care of patients.

Nursing is responsibility for the care of patients on a 24-hour basis. In order to maintain 24-hour coverage, seven days a week, there are three daily nursing shifts, usually a day shift, 7 A.M. to 3 P.M.; an evening shift, 3 P.M. to 11 P.M.; and a night shift, 11 P.M. to 7 A.M.

Other nursing service functions may include the general supervision of the *operating suite*, which consists of *operating rooms* (OR), storage, and associated space such as the *recovery room*, where patients stay immediately after the operation, under close supervision, before returning to their bed on the nursing unit. For obstetrical patients there are *labor rooms*, *delivery rooms*, and a *newborn nursery* with bassinets for the newborn babies. Maintenance of special cleanliness is vital in all these units and elaborate precautions are taken to prevent infections.

Nursing may include *Central Supply* (also called Central Medical and Surgical Supply, Central Sterile Supply), which washes, packages, and sterilizes (autoclaves) equipment, instruments, gowns, bandages, dressings, etc., primarily for the operating rooms, but also for all parts of the hospital where sterile materials are required. Central Supply may also be responsible for distribution of intravenous solutions (*I-V* fluids, to be injected in patients' veins).

Nursing education may include a hospital school of nursing (a *diploma school*) and *inservice nursing education*. Hospitals which do not have a school of nursing may provide clinical education for nursing students from nearby junior colleges, colleges, or universities for professional nurses (RNs) and for schools for practical nurses.

Ancillary Services

Clinical Services (Medical Services).   A number of medical services are hospital-based and may have physical space and hospital personnel working in it. These include:[10]

Anesthesiology.   This is a specialty of medicine concerned with the administration of local and general anesthetics, primarily in connection with surgery. This department may include *anesthesiologists* (who are physicians) and/or *nurse-anesthetists*, both of whom administer anesthesia.

Radiology.   This department is directed by a *radiologist* (who is a physician), using *X-rays* (or Roentgen rays) for the diagnosis (*diagnostic radiology*) and treatment (*radiation therapy*) of disease. The Department of Nuclear Medicine is sometimes associated with the Radiology Department. *Nuclear medicine* uses radioactive isotopes for the diagnosis and treatment of disease.

The Radiology Department requires a substantial amount of costly equipment and a physical space constructed so as to minimize the hazard of unwanted radiation exposure. A *radiographic technologist* (X-ray technician), who has a required high school education plus two years of training, takes the X-rays, which are then "read," or interpreted by the radiologist.

Pathology (Laboratories, Labs).   The hospital laboratories provide examination and analysis of tests on human tissue, bone, and excretions to aid in the diagnosis and treatment of patients. This is usually under the supervision of the hospital's pathologist-in-chief and, in a very large hospital, may include as many as 60 different sub-departments which do special types of analysis and related research. Major subcomponents include:

1. *The clinical laboratory*, which performs tests on blood, urine, bacteria, parasites, etc. Includes *hematology* (the study of blood); *biochemistry* (including the use of automatic analyzers); *bacteriology* (growth and identification of bacteria); *seriology* (antigen-antibody reactions, including the detection of syphilitic infections); *histology* (preparation of tissue removed during surgery); *cytology*

---

[10] Hospital-based physicians working full time within the hospital, particularly radiologists, anesthesiologists, pathologists, physiatrists, and emergency doctors may be paid in a number of different ways, including: (a) a salary from the hospital; (b) by directly billing patients for their services; (c) by a percentage of their department's gross income; (d) by a percentage of their department's net income; (e) a combination of these.

(preparation of body fluids to detect cell changes, such as those related to cancer).

2. *The anatomical laboratory* examines tissue both with the microscope and without (gross anatomy). *Autopsies* are performed here to determine the cause of death and a *morgue* for the dead is maintained.

Physical Medicine (Physiatry, Physical and Rehabilitative Medicine). Physiatry, Physical, and Rehabilitative Medicine (physical medicine, for short) are the same. Physical medicine is a specialty of medicine involved with the diagnosis and treatment of the disabled, convalescent, and physically handicapped patient, using heat, cold, exercise, water, etc., for therapy. *Physical therapists* assist the *physiatrist* (a medical doctor) in these tasks.

This department may also include *occupational therapy* and *speech therapy*. Occupational therapists help handicapped patients learn job-related skills and activities of daily living. Speech therapists help patients overcome speech problems. There are also corrective therapists, music therapists, and recreational therapists.

Outpatient Department (OPD). This department provides care for the nonemergency ambulatory patient, as contrasted with inpatient care. The department may be divided into numerous specialty clinics and may be staffed separately by doctors, nurses, clerks, etc.

Emergency Service (Emergency Room [ER], Emergency Department, Casualty Ward, Emergency Ward [EW]). This department provides immediate care around the clock for acutely ill patients coming to the hospital, although many of the patients using this service may not be acutely ill. There are a growing number of physicians who specialize in emergency medicine. Nurses, clerks, and other personnel may be assigned to this service. The hospital also may have an ambulance service.

Dental Service. This department provides dental care for ambulatory patients and sometimes for inpatients. The *dental staff* of the hospital, although smaller, is organized as part of the hospital's medical staff.

Some Other Professional and Therapeutic Services

The Pharmacy. This service usually purchases drugs and medications, maintains its supply, fills requisitions for the nursing *floor stock*, and fills prescriptions for individual patients. This department is run by the chief pharmacist; a drug and therapeutics committee provides a link with the medical staff. The hospital may maintain a *formulary*, which lists drugs that the medical staff finds acceptable for use in the hospital. It may list drugs by their generic names and permit the pharmacist to substitute between clinically similar drugs. This lowers the drug inventory and lowers the cost of drugs by allowing the pharmacist to purchase in bulk and to use low-cost generic name drugs.

The Blood Bank. This service maintains a supply of blood and blood derivatives such as plasma, for use in the hospital. In large hospitals there may be *organ banks* (e.g., an eye bank) which maintain a supply of human tissue and bone for replacement in other patients.

Electroencephalography (EEG). The EEG technician uses a machine (the electroencephalograph) to record the patient's brain waves with the use of electrodes attached to the patient's head. The recordings usually are interpreted by a physician to detect brain damage.

Electrocardiography. The EKG[11] (or ECG) technician uses machinery to record the electrical impulses produced by the heart muscles. These recordings are interpreted by a physician (often a cardiologist) to detect heart disease.

Inhalation Therapy. The inhalation therapist administers oxygen and therapeutic gas and mist inhalations to patients, at the direction of the patients' physicians, outside of the operating room.

Renal Dialysis Facility (Kidney Dialysis). The use of an artificial kidney machine.

Audiology (Audiologist, Speech Pathologist). The diagnosis and treatment of speech language problems.

Family Planning (birth control) services.

Home Care (Hospital-Based Home Care, Organized Home Care Program) provides care by doctors, nurses, social workers, therapists, etc., in the patient's home.

The Medical Records Department maintains, stores, and retrieves patient records and associated patient care statistics. A numbering

[11] EKG is derived from the original German spelling.

system is maintained for each patient and an index of patient names and record numbers is maintained to facilitate retrieval. Records are also indexed by disease, operation, and physician responsible for the patient. The records must be complete, signed by the doctor(s) responsible for the patient, and kept confidential so that only authorized personnel may see them. The *medical records librarian* in charge of this department supervises the file clerks, medical transcriptionists, and medical record technicians working in this department.

The Medical Library and the medical librarian in charge of it are not to be confused with the Medical Records Department and the medical record librarian (above). The Medical Library maintains scientific books and journals for the use of the medical staff and sometimes for other professional personnel.

Chaplaincy Service provides pastoral care and religious counseling for patients.

Social Service (Medical and Psychiatric Social Work) focuses on the social, economic, and environmental factors influencing the patient's condition. Knowledge of community resources is used to reduce the environmental and emotional obstacles to recovery, including financial support, post-hospital care (*discharge planning*), and working with the patient's family. Social Service often works very closely with psychiatry (psychiatric social work).

Dietary Services (the kitchen, inpatient food service cafeteria, food storage and purchasing, catering for special events, educational programs for dieticians, special diet kitchen, etc.). The Dietary Services Department may be headed by a *chief dietician* or a *food service manager*, or both. The education of dieticians emphasizes nutrition, the preparation of special diets, and the relationship between food and health. The background and education of food service managers emphasizes the production and management aspects of food preparation. A substantial number of patients may be on special diets (salt free, low fat, etc.) which must be prepared.

Administration

In addition to the administrator, his assistants, and associates, the administration of the hospital may include an *industrial engineer*, a *Data Processing Department* if the hospital has computer facilities, an *Employees' Health Clinic*, a front *Information Desk*, and other departments, some of which are described below.

Public Relations Department (PR). There may be a PR department to provide information about the hospital to the public, patients, and the press.

The Personnel Department recruits, interviews, and screens applicants for hospital positions and maintains salary scales. It keeps records of present and past hospital employees, orients new employees to the hospital, and maintains a position control system so that the complement of hospital jobs cannot be increased without approval of the administration. Personnel can perform many other functions, including *labor relations*, particularly if hospital personnel are unionized.

Fund-Raising may be a temporary or permanent department which solicits gifts and donations to the hospital, often in connection with the construction of new facilities.

Admissions (Admitting Office, Admitting Department) schedules patients for admission, keeps a waiting list, and a list of empty beds. The admissions personnel may assign patients to beds, and collect initial nonmedical information about the patient for the patient's record before he goes to his bed. They notify other parts of the hospital when the patient is admitted.

The Business Office produces patient bills, and collects money from patients and third party payers (accounts receivable). It maintains financial records, prepares budgets and cost reports for the hospital, and does the payroll for hospital employees.

Hospital Volunteers (Auxiliaries, Women's Auxiliary) are public-spirited citizens who donate their time to work for the hospital. They may help in a variety of tasks: escorting patients; arranging flowers; preparing bandages; running a gift shop, coffee shop, or thrift shop (which sells second-hand clothing, books, furniture, etc., and is located outside the hospital), with the proceeds donated to the hospital. Teenage girls who volunteer are often called *candy stripers*, because of the color of the uniforms they wear.

Support Services

Housekeeping is responsible for cleaning the hospital including floors, walls, and window-washing, and trash disposal.

Maintenance and Plant is often responsible for painting, repairs, carpentry, plumbing, the steam plant, electricity, air conditioning, elevators, fire alarm systems, emergency power sources, etc. There may be personnel assigned to maintain the hospital's *grounds* (ground crew), to run the *parking lot*, *print shop*, etc.

Purchasing and Stores is responsible for ordering supplies and equipment. It receives, stores, and delivers these items to the part of the hospital where they will be used. *Competitive bids* are sent out for high cost items and the hospital may participate with other hospitals in the area in a *joint purchasing program*, which can save money by purchasing in large volume.

Messenger and Transport Service delivers mail, supplies, and sometimes moves patients.

Laundry and Linen collects, sorts, washes, dries, presses, and repairs sheets, towels, gowns, uniforms, etc., for use in the hospital.

Telephone Switchboard receives incoming calls and maintains a *paging system* for reaching doctors in the hospital.

Some hospitals *contract* for services such as laundry, data processing, housekeeping, dietary, and others, with outside companies, or perform these services jointly with other hospitals (*shared services*).

Progressive Patient Care (PPC)

This is a way of dividing hospital patient services according to the severity of illness and the amount of care used by the patients. Hospitals have used all, part, or none of this system. Patient care levels, starting with the most intensive are:

1. *Intensive Care* (Intensive Care Unit; ICU), for severely ill patients needing a great deal of nursing care and close supervision. The severity of illness is similar in coronary care units (CCU), which treat patients with heart attacks.
2. *Intermediate Care*, for moderately ill patients.
3. *Self-Care*, for inpatients who can walk about, use a central dining area, and who can cope with activities of daily living.
4. *Long-Term Care (Extended Care Unit).*
5. *Home Care* (Hospital-based Home Care, Organized Home Care Program; in contrast to a doctor's home visit), the organized provision of care in the patient's home by nurses, therapists, social workers, physicians, etc.

The Flow of Work in a Community General Hospital

Another way to conceptualize the activities in a community general hospital is to track the events associated with a patient's admission, diagnostic work-up, treatment, and discharge. In Table 1–2 this is

Table 1–2.   Part I
The Progress of a Herniorrhaphy Patient Through A Community General Hospital

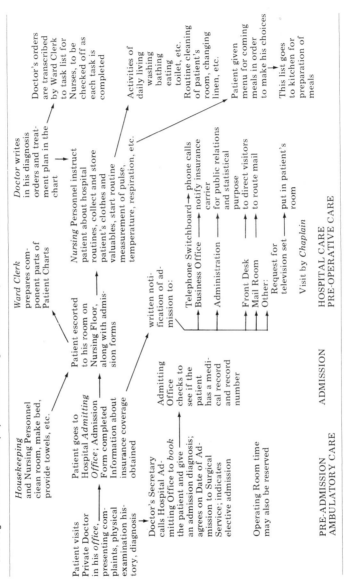

Housekeeping and Nursing Personnel clean room, make bed, provide towels, etc.

Ward Clerk prepares component parts of Patient Charts

Doctor writes in his diagnosis orders and treatment plan in the chart

Nursing Personnel instruct patient about hospital routines, collect and store patient's clothes and valuables, start routine measurement of pulse, temperature, respiration, etc.

Doctor's orders are transcribed by Ward Clerk to task list for Nurses, to be checked off as each task is completed

Activities of daily living
washing
bathing
eating
toilet, etc.
Routine cleaning of patient's room, changing linen, etc.

Patient given menu for coming meals in order to make his choices

This list goes to kitchen for preparation of meals

Patient escorted to his room on Nursing Floor, along with admission forms

written notification of admission to:

Telephone Switchboard → phone calls
Business Office → notify insurance carrier
Administration → for public relations and statistical purpose
Front Desk → to direct visitors
Mail Room → to route mail
Other:
Request for television set → put in patient's room

Visit by *Chaplain*

Patient goes to Hospital *Admitting Office*; Admission Form completed Information about insurance coverage obtained

Admitting Office checks to see if the patient has a medical record and record number

Patient visits Private Doctor in his *office*, presenting complaints, physical examination history, diagnosis

Doctor's Secretary calls Hospital Admitting Office to *book* the patient and give an admission diagnosis; agrees on Date of Admission to Surgical Service; indicates elective admission

Operating Room time may also be reserved

PRE-ADMISSION AMBULATORY CARE

ADMISSION

HOSPITAL CARE PRE-OPERATIVE CARE

Table 1-2. Part II

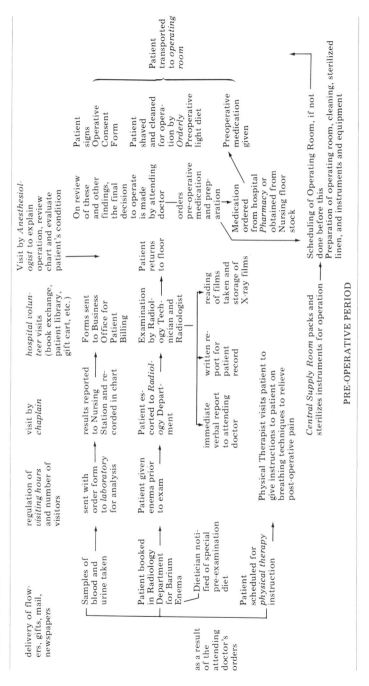

Table 1-2.   Part III
The Progress of a Herniorrhaphy Patient Through a Community General Hospital

Operation
Administration of Anesthesia
Operative team of Surgeon
Surgical Nurse
Surgical Technicians
Elaborate precautions to maintain sterile operating room environment

→ Patient removed to *Recovery Room* for several hours under supervision of Operating Suite Nurses and Anesthesiologist

→ Patient returned to room on Nursing Floor and regular nursing coverage

Daily Routines Continue
Change of Dressings
Help in early ambulation

Discharge Planning by Nursing and *Social Service* (This is important for some patients who need special transportation, home care or placement in a nursing home, which is often necessary for hernia patients)

Doctor's Discharge Note in Medical Record

Day of Discharge
Return of Patient's Belongings
Check out at Business Office for completion of Insurance forms and payment plan
Patient Goes Home

Patient Chart sent to *Medical Records* Department
Reviewed for completeness
Abstract data for patient statistics
Transcribing discharge summary and diagnosis

Patient returns to Doctor's office for removal of stitches and follow-up care, if necessary

Business Office calculates patient's bill, based on services used
→ Form sent to insurer for payment
→ Bill sent to patient for payment (*credit and collections department*)

OPERATION AND RECOVERY ROOM   POST-OPERATIVE PERIOD   DISCHARGE   POST-HOSPITALIZATION AMBULATORY CARE

done for a patient requiring an uncomplicated elective hernia operation. This operation, called a herniorrhaphy, is one of the most frequent reasons for hospital admission and is not considered a complex or particularly difficult operation. As the table shows, even this routine admission requires the coordinated activities of a large number of different people and departments. Not all hospital personnel are directly involved with every patient and, therefore, only some are included in this table. Other patients would call for the involvement of other types of personnel.

Although this general outline is fairly typical, the details will vary from patient to patient and from hospital to hospital.

References

Robert M. Sloane and Beverly L. Sloane, *A Guide to Health Facilities Personnel and Management*, (St. Louis: C.V. Mosby Co., 1971).

U.S. Department of Labor, Manpower Administration, *Job Description and Organizational Analysis for Hospitals and Related Health Services.* Revised Edition. (Washington, D.C.: U.S. Government Printing Office, 1971.)

John R. McGibony, *Principles of Hospital Administration*, Second Edition, (New York: G.P. Putnam's Sons, 1969).

Joseph K. Owen, *Modern Concepts of Hospital Administration*, (Philadelphia: W.B. Saunders, Co., 1962).

American Hospital Association, *Cumulative Guide to Hospital Literature*, (Chicago: The American Hospital Association, Quarterly).

6. LICENSURE, CERTIFICATION, REGISTRATION AND ACCREDITATION OF HEALTH FACILITIES

Licensure. An agency of government, usually at the state level, grants permission to an institution with specified characteristics to perform a defined set of functions.

The following facilities and services are licensed in one or more states plus the District of Columbia. (1973)*

General Hospitals (50 states), Homes for Dependent Children (48), Homes for Unwed Mothers (44), Facilities for Handicapped Children

*Health Resources Statistics, 1974. National Center for Health Statistics, U.S. Department of HEW, PHS, HSMHA (Rockville, Maryland), 1974.

(16), Hospitals for Mentally Retarded (42), Nursing Homes (51), Facilities for Emotionally Disturbed Children (33), Specialty Hospitals (51), Ambulance Services (27), Blood Banks (7), Clinical Laboratories (25), Home Health Services (7), Medical Group Practices (1), Opticianry Establishments (3), and Pharmacies (51).

Most licensing agencies are within Health and Welfare Departments of state government.

Certification. Health Facilities participating in the Medicare and Medicaid Programs must be certified by designated state agencies. These include hospitals, nursing homes, home health agencies and independent laboratories.

Registration. The American Hospital Association maintains a system of registration of hospitals in the United States. This list is published yearly in the *AHA Guide Issue.* The National Center for Health Statistics keeps an inventory of inpatient facilities called the *Master Facility Inventory* (MFI).

Accreditation programs are voluntary non-government evaluations of health care facilities which choose to participate. The best known of these is the *Joint Commission on Accreditation of Hospitals* (JCAH). The JCAH had its origin with Dr. Ernest Amory Codman's interest in evaluating the end-results of hospital care, and the American College of Surgeons (ACS) concern for surgical competence, and the quality of hospital medical records. The ACS started accrediting hospitals in 1918. This effort evolved into the JCAH which was formed in 1951 as a joint effort of the American College of Surgeons, American College of Physicians, American Hospital Association (AHA), American Medical Association (AMA), and the Canadian Medical Association. The Canadians withdrew in 1959 to found their own accrediting body.

For a hospital to be accredited by the JCAH, it must be accepted for registration by the AHA, ask for an accreditation survey by a JCAH survey team, and pay a fee. The hospital is either accredited for 3 years, 1 year, or unaccredited. The JCAH develops standards of acceptable practices and provides advice to hospitals about these practices.

In 1966, the JCAH formed the *Accreditation Council for Long Term Care Facilities*, a joint effort of the American Association of Homes for the Aging, AHA, AMA, and the American Nursing Home Association.

In 1969, the JCAH formed the *Accreditation Council for Facilities for the Mentally Retarded* (Council Members are: American Academy of Pediatrics, American Association of Mental Deficiency, American Nurses Association (ANA), American Psychiatric Association, American Psychological Association, National Association for Retarded Citizens, National Association of Private Residential Facilities for the Mentally Retarded, and United Cerebral Palsy Association.)

In 1970, the JCAH formed the *Accreditation Council for Psychiatric Facilities.* (Council members are: American Academy of Child Psychiatry, American Association of Mental Deficiency, American Association of Psychiatric Services for Children, AHA, American Psychiatric Association, Association of Mental Health Administrators, National Association of Private Psychiatric Hospitals, National Association of State Mental Health Program Directors and National Council of Community Mental Health Centers.)

The JCAH is undertaking an accreditation program for Neighborhood Health Centers.

Other Accrediting Programs cover:

- Community Nursing Services (Program sponsored by the National League for Nursing (NLN) and the American Public Health Association (APHA).
- Clinical Laboratories (Commission on Laboratory Inspection and Accreditation of the American College of Pathologists)
- Rehabilitation Facilities (Commission on Accreditation of Rehabilitation Facilities (CARF).) Members are the Association of Rehabilitation Centers, National Association of Sheltered Workshops and Homebound Programs, AHA, Goodwill Industries of America, National Association of Hearing and Speech Agencies, National Easter Seal Society for Crippled Children and Adults, and the National Rehabilitation Association.
- Blood Banks: American Association of Blood Banks (AABB)
- Medical Group Practice: American Association of Medical Clinics (AAMC)

In addition, the American Osteopathic Association (AOA) accredits osteopathic hospitals and extended care facilities. The AOA annually publishes a registry of Accredited Osteopathic Institutions.

7. INSTITUTIONALIZED PERSONS

Table 1–3 shows the location of the 1.7 million people who were were found to be residents in Health Institutions at the time of the

Table 1-3. Number of Institutionalized Persons 1970 (Resident Populations in Health Institutions)

Total	1,721,970
All Mental Hospitals and Residential Treatment Centers	433,890
Tuberculosis Hospitals	16,912
Chronic Disease Hospitals	67,120
Homes for the Aged and Dependent	927,514
Homes and Schools for the Mentally Handicapped	201,992
Homes for the Dependent and Neglected Children	47,594
Homes and Schools for the Physically Handicapped	
For the Blind	6,949
For the Deaf	8,911
Other	6,879
Homes for Unwed Mothers	4,209

Source: U.S. Government, Department of Health, Education, and Welfare, National Center for Health Statistics. *Health United States 1975*, p. 315.

1970 U.S. census. The largest group of these people are to be found in nursing homes.

8. NURSING HOMES

Prior to 1930 there were very few nursing homes. The Social Security Act of 1935, by making money available to the elderly beneficiaries, encouraged the growth of proprietary boarding and nursing homes and the decline of public alms houses serving the indigent.

Medicare and Medicaid provided further impetus to the growth of nursing homes. All states license nursing homes, not all of which participate in Medicare or Medicaid. In 1966 the JCAH assumed responsibility for the voluntary accreditation of extended care, nursing care, and resident care facilities.

Today almost one in twenty Americans 65 years old and older occupies a bed in a nursing or related home. About 90 percent of nursing home patients are over 65. The majority of nursing homes are proprietary. Nursing homes are licensed by the state and, in addition, are usually certified for participation in Medicare and Medicaid.

There is no agreed upon set of definitions to define the different types of nursing homes.

The National Center for Health Statistics classifies and defines nursing homes as follows:

They are classified according to the predominate service provided.

A *nursing care home* has 50 percent or more of the residents receiving one or more nursing services and the facility has at least one registered nurse (RN) or licensed practical nurse (LPN), employed 35 or more hours a week. Nursing services include nasal feeding, catheterization, irrigation, oxygen therapy, full bed bath, enema, hypodermic injection, intravenous injection, temperature-pulse-respiration, blood pressure, application of dressing or bandage, or bowel and bladder retraining.

A *personal care home with nursing care* is defined as one in which either: (a) some, but less, than 50 percent of the residents receive nursing care or (b) more than 50% of the residents receive nursing care, but no RNs or LPNs are employed full time on the staff.

A *personal care home without nursing care* routinely provides three or more of the following personal services, but no nursing service. Personal services include: rub or massage service, or assistance with bathing, dressing, correspondence or shopping, walking or getting about, or eating.

A *domiciliary care home* routinely provides less than three personal services as described above and no nursing service. This type of facility provides a sheltered environment primarily for persons who are able to care for themselves.

Source: *Health Resources Statistics, 1974*, p. 340.

Today the ECF is no longer a distinct classification of facility, but has been merged into the category of Skilled Nurse Facility (SNF). In addition to the three levels of SNF, ICF (Intermediate Care Facility), and Residential Facility, the states may define four levels of nursing home care. The higher the level of care, the greater the care needs of the patient and the higher the level of reimbursement from Medicaid.

SNFs provide continuous nursing service on a 24-hour basis. Registered nurses, licensed practical nurses, and nursing aides provide services prescribed by the patient's physician. The emphasis is on medical nursing care with restorative therapy, physical therapy, occupational therapy, etc. Medicare and Medicaid pay for care in SNFs. Medicare will pay if

• the home is certified as a SNF;

- the patient has spent at least three consecutive days in a hospital and is admitted to the SNF within 14 days after discharge;
- the patient's physician says the care is needed for the illness for which the patient has been hospitalized;
- skilled nursing care and rehabilitative services as defined by the Social Security Administration are required by the patient on a daily basis.

Medicare pays for the first twenty days and for part of the next eighty days, if the patient qualifies. A utilization review mechanism is required.

Unlike Medicare, Medicaid program benefits vary from state to state. Medicare does not provide ICF benefits, but Medicaid does.

The intermediate care facility is intended as a less expensive alternative to the skilled nursing home in the same way that the skilled nursing home is intended as a substitute for the more expensive hospital.

Three associations represent nursing homes. The American Nursing Home Association (the largest, representing profit and not-for-profit homes), the American Association of Homes for the Aging (represents only non-profit homes), and the National Council of Health Care Services (large for-profit nursing home chains). In addition, there are 300 national organizations representing the elderly.

Three types of services are offered in nursing homes. These are:

1. *Nursing care:* by RNs and LPNs. Also physical therapy, occupational therapy, dental services, dietary consultations, lab, X-ray services, and a pharmaceutical dispensary
2. *Personal care:* help in walking, getting in and out of bed, bathing, dressing and eating, preparation of special diets prescribed by a physician
3. *Residential care:* room and board in a protective environment and a planned program for the residents' social and spiritual needs.

Nursing homes vary according to services provided, from those with extensive nursing and other services (including full-time physicians), personal care homes with and without nursing, domiciliary homes (homes for the aged), and special housing for the aged.[12]

Licensure of *nursing home administrators* (SNFs, ICFs) is mandatory in all states. Licensure requires 15 hours a year of continuing education.

[12] The "aged," the "elderly," "old people," "senior citizens," and "golden age groups" are used interchangeably for people 65 years old and over.

9. OTHER HEALTH SERVICES

Ambulance Services. Emergency ambulance services are provided by police departments, fire departments, volunteer community groups, welfare departments, morticians, hospitals, taxi companies, gasoline service stations and commercial ambulance companies. They use a variety of vehicles, from completely equipped modern ambulances to station wagons and trucks.

About 40% of the country's 14,100 ambulance services (25,900 vehicles) are provided by funeral homes. There are about 207,000 ambulance personnel.

Blood Banks. The American Association of Blood Banks (AABB) defines a blood bank as a medical facility that recruits at least 100 donors per year, draws, processes, stores, and distributes human whole blood, and its derivatives. They include:

- Hospital Blood Bank (Primarily for its own needs. If the hospital only receives its blood from other Blood Banks, it has a transfusion service.)
- Community Blood Bank. (A non-profit facility to serve the needs of a number of hospitals in the area.)
- Regional Centers of the American National Red Cross (59 Centers)
- Other Blood Programs (For-profit blood banks)

Of the 5,400 blood banks, most are in hospitals. The Bureau of Biologics of the Food and Drug Administration (FDA) licenses the largest 530 blood bank facilities accounting for 80% of the U.S. blood supply.

Clinical (Medical) Laboratories carry out tests on specimens from the human body to detect the presence, absence or extent of disease. They may be physically located in a doctor's office, group practice, hospital, public health agency, or as a privately owned corporation. An independent lab may operate under the direction of a physician or other scientist. There are 12,300 laboratories in the country (1971).

Medicare certifies 2,900 independent labs (independent of attending consulting doctor's office or hospitals).

The Clinical Laboratories Improvement Act of 1967 (Pl 90-174) provides for Federal Licensure of clinical laboratories involved in interstate commerce.

Dental Laboratories fabricate dentures and other dental appliances; by 1971 there were an estimated 9,900 commercial dental laboratories in the U.S.; 4,400 in dentists' private practice offices, 800 in institutions, and the rest are independent commercial labs.

Opticianry Establishments. The American Board of Opticianry defines opticianry as the art and science of optics as applied to the compounding, filling and adapting of ophthalmic prescriptions, products, and accessories. Opticianry establishments primarily sell eyeglasses and related optical goods. In 1969, there were 11,000 dispensing opticians and contact lens technicians, and 5,900 opticianry establishments.

Rehabilitation Facilities provide services for the restoration of the disabled to physical, mental, social, vocational and economic usefulness, including speech and hearing centers, sheltered workshops, evaluation units, and comprehensive rehabilitation centers (either free-standing or part of a larger medical complex). There are about 3,000 such facilities which have relationships to State rehabilitation agencies.

Table 1-5-1-9 provide some basic data on hospitals, nursing homes, and other inpatient services.

10. REGULATION OF HEALTH SERVICES INSTITUTIONS

Regulation, broadly defined, can be classified as *governmental* and *voluntary*. Regulation can be internal or external to the organization. It can be done by professionals collectively, or it can be done by consumers and laymen. It can be achieved through voice or exit[13] (see Table 1-10 and section on "Quality Control").

Health organizations regulate the performance of their personnel through *administrative policies and procedures.* In addition, the professionals who practice in organizational settings abide by collectively defined rules and by-laws, and by *peer review* of performance. Organizations may elect to abide by the recommended policies of external accrediting agencies, such as *voluntary planning groups*, the JCAH, and educational accrediting groups. An important part of professional education is the internalizing of ethical values which

[13] Albert O. Hirschman, *Exit Voice and Loyalty* (Cambridge, Mass.: Harvard University Press, 1970).

Table 1-4. Classifications of Nursing Homes*

Medicare–Medicaid Definitions 1965–1974	Medicare–Medicaid Definitions 1974–	National Center for Health Statistics** 1974	U.S. Government 1973***
Skilled Nursing Home (SNF)	Skilled Nursing Facility (SNF)	Nursing Care Home	Nursing I Facilities
Extended Care Facility (ECF)			
Intermediate Care Facility (ICF)	Intermediate Care Facility (ICF)	Personal Care Home with Nursing Care	Nursing II Facilities
		Personal Care Home without Nursing Care	Residential Facilities
	Residential Facility (Rest Home)	Domiciliary Care Home	

(These two definitions are comparable.)

*Also called, Home for the Aged, Old Age Institutions. These are Multilevel Facilities.
**Health Resources Statistics, 1974. National Center for Health Statistics, U.S. Department of HEW, PHS, HSMHA (Rockville, Maryland), 1974.
***U.S. Department of Health, Education and Welfare. *Nursing Homes: A County and Metropolitan Area Data Book 1973.*
See: B.B. Manard, C. Skait, D.W.L. VanGils. *Old Age Institutions.* (Lexington, Massachusetts: Lexington Books, 1975)

Table 1-5. Hospitals and Hospital Beds: Selected Years 1963 through 1973

Year	Total hospitals	General medical and surgical	Specialty				
			Total	Psychiatric	Geriatric and chronic	Tuberculosis	Other[1]
Facilities							
1972	7,481	6,491	990	497	78	75	340
1970	7,638	6,574	1,064	494	126	108	336
1967	8,147	6,685	1,462	573	333	169	387
1963	8,183	6,710	1,473	581	211	258	423
Beds							
1973	1,449,062	1,030,432	418,630	338,574	22,350	10,215	47,491
1970	1,534,779	1,004,415	530,364	437,969	38,144	19,836	34,415
1967	1,631,101	958,729	672,372	545,913	61,211	33,335	31,913
1963	1,549,952	811,876	738,076	614,104	38,213	50,075	35,685
Beds per 1,000 population							
1973	6.9	4.9	2.0	1.6	0.1	0.05	0.2
1970	7.6	5.0	2.6	2.2	0.2	0.1	0.2
1967	8.3	4.9	3.4	2.8	0.3	0.2	0.2
1963	8.3	4.3	4.0	3.3	0.2	0.3	0.2

1. Includes eye, ear, nose, and throat hospitals; epileptic hospitals; alcoholic hospitals; narcotic hospitals; maternity hospitals; orthopedic hospitals; physical rehabilitation hospitals and other hospitals.

Source: Health Resources Statistics, 1974. National Center for Health Statistics, USDHEW, PHS, HSMHA (Rockville, Maryland).

From: Unpublished data from the National Center for Health Statistics master facility census. National Center for Health Statistics: *Health Resources Statistics,* 1969. PHS Pub. 1509. Public Health Service, U.S. Department of Health, Education and Welfare. Washington. U.S. Government Printing Office, May 1970. U.S. Bureau of the Census: *Current Population Reports.* Series P-25, No. 462, June 1971. National Center for Health Statistics, *Health United States, 1975,* DHEW Pub. HRA 76-1232, Washington, D.C.

Table 1-6. Ownership of Hospitals: 1972

Ownership	Total Hospitals	General medical and surgical	Specialty				
			Total	Psychiatric	Chronic Disease	Tuberculosis	Other[1]
Total	7,481	6,491	990	497	78	75	340
Government	2,770	2,248	522	328	49	70	75
Federal	405	369	36	29	—	—	7
State-Local	2,365	1,879	486	299	49	70	68
Proprietary	986	811	175	88	8	—	79
Non-Profit	3,725	3,432	293	81	21	5	186
Church	854	797	57	14	5	1	37
Other	2,871	2,635	236	67	16	4	149

1. Includes eye, ear, nose, and throat hospitals; epileptic hospitals, alcoholic hospitals; narcotic hospitals; maternity hospitals; orthopedic hospitals; physical rehabilitation hospitals; and other hospitals.

Source: Health Resource Statistics, 1974. National Center for Health Statistics, USDHEW, PHS, HSMHA (Rockville, Maryland), p. 365.

Table 1-7. Ownership of Nursing Care and Related Homes: 1971

Ownership	Total Homes	Nursing Care	Personal Care Homes		Domiciliary Care
			With Nursing	Without Nursing	
Number of Homes					
Total Homes	22,004	12,871	3,568	5,369	196
Government	1,368	872	223	265	8
Federal	67	18	18	28	3
State-Local	1,301	854	205	237	5
Proprietary	17,049	9,963	2,317	4,611	158
Non-Profit	3,587	2,036	1,028	493	30
Church	912	500	307	99	6
Other	2,675	1,536	721	394	24
Number of Beds					
Total Beds	1,201,598	917,707	192,347	88,317	3,227
Government	122,972	91,708	23,658	7,466	140
Federal	5,764	1,557	2,383	1,733	91
State-Local	117,208	90,151	21,275	5,733	49
Proprietary	803,696	663,031	73,442	65,845	1,378
Non-Profit	274,930	162,968	95,247	15,006	1,709
Church	81,336	43,655	33,215	3,713	753
Other	193,594	119,313	62,032	11,293	956

Source: Health Resources Statistics, 1974. National Center for Health Statistics, USDHEW, PHS, HSMHA (Rockville, Maryland), p. 394.

Table 1-8.   Inpatient Health Facilities: Selected Years 1963 through 1972

Type of Facility	1963	1967	1971	1972
Total Facilities	27,171	30,586	34,451	—
Hospitals	8,183	8,147	7,678	7,481
General Medical and Surgical Hospitals	6,710	6,685	6,607	6,491
Specialty Hospitals	1,473	1,462	1,071	990
Psychiatric	581	573	533	497
Geriatric[1] and Chronic	211	333	90	78
Tuberculosis	258	169	99	75
Other[2]	423	387	349	340
Nursing Care and Related Homes	16,701	19,141	22,004	—
Nursing Care	8,128	10,636	12,871	—
Personal Care Home with Nursing	4,958	3,853	3,568	—
Personal Care Home without Nursing	2,927	4,396	5,369	—
Domiciliary Care	688	256	196	—
Other Inpatient Health Facilities	2,287	3,298	4,769	—

1. 1963 and 1967—Geriatric and Chronic. 1971 and 1972—Chronic Only.
2. Includes eye, ear, nose and throat hospitals; epileptic hospitals; alcoholic hospitals; narcotic hospitals; maternity hospitals; orthopedic hospitals; physical rehabilitation hospitals; and other hospitals.
Source: Health Resources Statistics, 1974. National Center for Health Statistics, USDHEW, PHS, HSMHA (Rockville, Maryland), p. 345.

enjoin the professional to strive for high ideals of public service and a commitment to excellence. The AMA has developed such a Code of Medical Ethics for physicians. To the extent that these ethical ideals are internalized, they are a form of professional self-regulation.

Public, Lay, or Consumer Regulation

The *public* are all people, whether or not they are receiving care.

A *layman* is a nonprofessional; as in "a lay board of trustees."

A *consumer* is a *patient*, a recipient of care, or a purchaser of a health-related product. Public regulation is derived either through "exit," that is, choice in the market place, or "voice," that is, speaking out about their preferences. Part of the aim of public regulations is often to promote and encourage organizational and professional self-regulation.

Exit (*"Free choice of physician"*) refers to the idea that patients should have a choice of physician. *Dual Choice* is usually used in the

Table 1-9. Beds in Inpatient Health Facilities: Selected Years 1963 through 1972

Type of Facility	Number				Number per 1,000 Population			
	1963	1967	1971	1972	1963	1967	1971	1972
Total Beds	2,448,512	2,871,655	3,194,213	—	13.1	14.7	15.9	—
Hospitals	1,549,952	1,631,010	1,507,988	1,467,040	8.3	8.3	7.4	7.0
General Medical and Surgical Hospitals	811,876	958,729	1,004,799	1,014,064	4.3	4.9	4.9	4.9
Specialty Hospitals	738,076	672,372	503,189	452,976	4.0	3.4	2.5	2.2
Psychiatric	614,104	545,913	418,487	372,603	3.3	2.8	2.0	1.8
Geriatric and Chronic	38,213	61,211	24,614	23,962	0.2	0.3	0.1	0.1
Tuberculosis	50,074	33,335	17,806	12,351	0.3	0.2	0.1	0.1
Other	35,685	31,913	42,282	44,060	0.2	0.2	0.2	0.2
Nursing Care and Related Homes	568,560	836,554	1,201,598	—	3.0	4.3	5.9	—
Nursing Care	319,224	584,052	917,707	—	1.7	3.0	4.5	—
Personal Care Home with Nursing	188,306	181,096	192,347	—	1.0	0.9	0.9	—
Personal Care Home without Nursing	48,962	66,787	88,317	—	0.3	0.3	0.4	—
Domiciliary Care	12,068	4,619	3,227	—	0.1	0.0	0.2	—
Other Inpatient Health Facilities	330,000	404,000	484,627	—	1.8	2.1	2.4	—

Source: Health Resources Statistics, 1974, National Center for Health Statistics, U.S. Department of HEW, PHS, HSMHA (Rockville, Maryland), 1974, p. 346.

Table 1-10.   Typology of Regulation

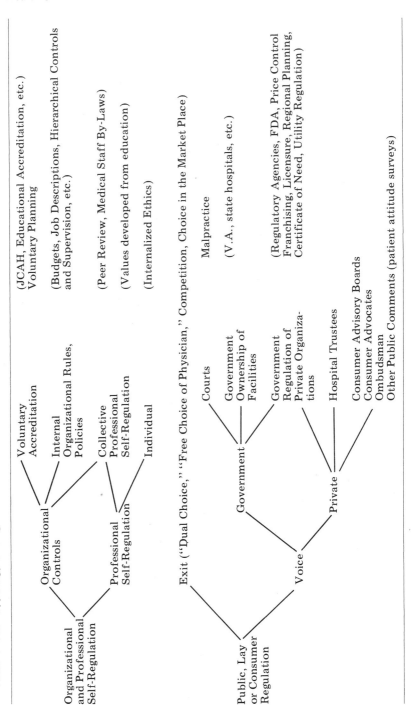

context of HMO's and PGP's, where the insured person has a choice of either the HMO or insurance coverage which will pay for the non-plan doctor and hospital of his choice.

Voice can be through government or private channels. The former includes redress from *malpractice* through the courts, government ownership and operation of health services, and government regulation of private organizations, some of which are described below. Private channels include (lay) *boards of trustees* which have direct responsibility for the operation of the organization, and *consumer advisory boards* which serve in an advisory capacity. An *ombudsman* is an employee of an organization (public or private) who is responsible for channeling patient complaints and helping resolve problems that arise this way. A *consumer advocate* acts as an ombudsman, but may or may not be employed by a health delivery organization. In addition, public comments may be elicited systematically through *patient attitude surveys*, or may be initiated by patients in an informal way.

The influence of these regulatory mechanisms will vary from organization to organization and there is no consensus as to their relative impact on the delivery of health services.

Government Regulation of Health Institutions is primarily at the state level, with some exceptions at the federal level, such as the *FDA*, and the *Price Control Commission* which regulates allowable price increases.

Licensure. Hospitals, nursing homes, pharmacies, and sometimes other facilities such as clinics are licensed by the state. They are periodically inspected to insure that they meet minimum standards. In addition, health facilities, like non-health-related buildings, are subject to a variety of inspections for *fire safety, building codes, zoning regulations, boiler* and *elevator performance,* ¿tc.

Institutional Licensure is a concept which is nowhere in actual practice. Instead of licensing doctors, nurses, and other professionals who work in an organization, the organization itself would be licensed so that the personnel working within the organization would be exempt from professional licensure. Then, for example, nurses would be allowed to perform tasks in the organization which are ordinarily restricted to physicians. The idea is that there would be more flexibility and substitution with respect to who does what. It would also minimize *blocked mobility*, in other words, the opportunity for an LPN to do the work of an RN, and an RN to do the work of an M.D.

Certificate of Need Laws.   About half the states have such laws to the effect that no health facility can spend more than some specified amount (say, $100,000) on a new construction without state approval. The facility must justify to the state agency that the construction is needed and will not duplicate existing facilities (*duplication of services*).

Franchising. The state establishes conditions under which the hospital or other providor may do business. This idea comes from franchising in business.

Utility Regulation proposes that facilities be regulated by a regulatory board or agency, appointed or controlled by the state, which has the power to approve budgets, prices, expansion, profits, and scope of services provided, in the same way that other utilities (such as electrical and telephone companies) are now regulated.

Health Authority. The creation of a single state organization which controls all licensure of facilities and personnel, and regulation of health insurance, and which channels state and federal funds to private health organizations. This follows the model of port and airport authorities.

Regionalization is the concept that health facilities should be responsible for geographically-defined populations and that there should be systematic relationships and referral patterns between different facilities. For example, there might be "front line" clinics for *primary ambulatory care* linked to community hospitals for *secondary care.* The community hospitals would be linked to medical centers or referral hospitals (*tertiary care*) for very specialized care. This example can be shown diagrammatically as follows:

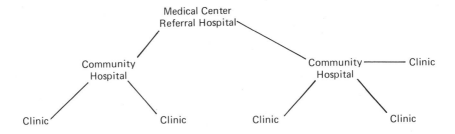

Nursing homes and other facilities could also be included. As such, regionalization is a concept for the flow of patients and location of services, rather than regulation per se. This concept is transformed into regulation via *Regional Planning.* Regional planning originally started on a voluntary basis for hospitals. This has been largely superceded by the Comprehensive Health Planning and Public Health Amendments of 1966 (PL 89-749). This law created *local health planning agencies* called *314-B Agencies* or *B agencies*, and *statewide health planning agencies* called *314-A Agencies* or *A agencies.* (314-A and 314-B are the relevant paragraphs in PL 89-749.) This was followed by the Health Planning and Resources Development Act of 1974 (PL 93-641) which created local Health Services Areas associated with Health Services Agencies (HSA's) responsible for health planning and development. It also supported State Health Planning and Development Agencies.

The HSA's are required to gather and analyze data and develop health systems plans (HSP's) for long-term objectives and annual implementation plans (AIP's), to coordinate activities with PSRO's review, and approve or disapprove applications for federal funds, review proposed capital expenditures, estimate needs for new services, and recommend projects for modernizing, constructing and converting health facilities in the area.

Chapter 2

Health Manpower

1. PERSONNEL AND PROFESSIONS IN THE HEALTH FIELD

Professional, Paraprofessional, Subprofessional, Semiprofessional. The word professional has no consistent or agreed upon meaning. Most occupational groups in the health field aspire to being considered professions. There are a number of component parts to the definition of a profession.[1]

1. Formal education and examination are required for membership in the profession.
2. Certification or licensure is required for membership, reflecting community sanction or approval.
3. The existence of regional or national associations.
4. There is a code of ethics.
5. There is a body of systematic scientific knowledge and technical skill required.
6. The members function with a degree of autonomy and authority, under the assumption that they alone have the expertise to make decisions in their area of competence.

Medicine is often considered the occupation which most closely approaches the prototype of a profession.

[1] See Ernest Greenwood, "Attributes of a Profession," p. 206 in Sigmund Nosow and William H. Form (editors), *Man, Work, and Society* (New York: Basic Books, 1962) and Eliot Freidson, *Profession of Medicine* (New York: Dodd Mead & Co., 1970).

Paraprofessional or *ancillary personnel* refer to those who work alongside a professional; *subprofessional* refers to occupations which are subordinate to other professions; and *semiprofessionals* do not have all the characteristics of a profession.[2] *Allied* health personnel are those who work with physicians; this category usually includes all hospital personnel, but excludes, for example, chiropractors.

Registration, Certification and Licensure

Registration is the process by which qualified individuals are listed on an official roster maintained by a governmental or non-governmental agency. Registration in some cases allows the individual to use a designation after his or her name. For example, a cytotechnologist registered by the Board of Registry of the American Society of Clinical Pathologists may use the designation CT (ASCP).

Certification is the process by which a non-governmental agency or association grants recognition to an individual who has not certain predetermined qualifications specified by that agency or association. A *diplomate* is one certified by an agency recognized as professionally competent to grant such certification.

Licensure is the process by which an agency of government grants permission to persons meeting predetermined qualifications to engage in a given occupation and/or use a particular title. Legislation usually establishes educational experience and personal qualifications, requires successful completion of an examination and provides issuance of a license as a prior condition for entrance into the occupation.*

As of 1973, over 30 health professions were licensed in one or more states. Licensed in all states are dental hygienists, dentists, embalmers, environmental health engineers, optometrists, pharmacists, physical therapists, medical and osteopathic physicians, podiatrists, practical and registered nurses and veterinarians. Some states license nursing home administrator (49 states), clinical laboratory director (19), medical technologist (10), dental laboratory technician (1), funeral director (44), midwife (23), nurse midwife (7),

---

[2] Etzioni, Amitai (editor), *The Semi-Professions and Their Organization* (The Free Press, 1961). The ill-defined word *ancillary personnel* is also used here.

Health Resources Statistics, 1974. National Center for Health Statistics, U.S. Department of HEW, PHS, HSMHA (Rockville, Maryland), 1974.

ophthalmic laboratory technician (2), optician (17), physical therapy assistant (14), physician's assistant (1), psychiatric aide (3), psychologist (47), radiologic technologist (3), respiratory therapist (1), sanitarian (35), sanitarian technician (1), social worker (11), speech pathologist and audiologist (14). Chiropractors are licensed in 49 states.

The terms technologist, therapist, technician, assistant and aide are now used in no systematic way. The following definitions are suggested:[3]

Technologist Therapist	This occupation requires education at, or above, the baccalaureate level
Technician Assistant	Requires education at, or beyond, the two-year college level (the Associate Degree level) after high school
Aide	Requires less than two years beyond high school or on-the-job training

In the sections that follow there will be more space devoted to physicians, dentists, and nurses because these health occupations are most frequently referred to, and their education is often used as a foil or mirror to compare with that of other professional groups.

Accreditation of Educational Programs for Health Professionals

Accreditation is a means of non-governmental evaluation of educational institutions. Accreditation can be concerned with an institution as a whole or a specialized part of an institution.

The U.S. Commissioner of Education publishes a list of recognized accrediting agencies for the purpose of determining institutional eligibility for Federal Programs of assistance.

Otherwise, the Federal government does not exercise control over private educational institutions. State control varies substantially and, in general, private institutions of higher education function with considerable autonomy.

The National Commission on Accreditation is a private, independent agency whose members include colleges and universities which grants recognition to qualified, voluntary accrediting agencies. In the health

[3] *Health Resources Statistics* HEW, HSMHA, February 1972.

field, the *Council on Medical Education* of the American Medical Association (AMA), plays the major role in accrediting educational programs. Jointly with the Association of American Medical Colleges (AAMC), it accredits medical schools and with 28 collaborating organizations, the Council on Medical Education accredits educational programs for 24 allied health occupations. (See Table 2-3)

Diagram 2-1 summarizes the entrance of a person into a health profession starting with education, licensure, certification and/or registration and place of practice or employment. It shows the role of accreditation and licensure of institutions and educational programs.

Health Professions and Occupations

There are over two hundred occupations in the health field and new ones are constantly appearing. Table 2-1 lists some of these occupations. Table 2-2 estimates the total number of personnel within selected health care occupations. Table 2-3 lists those agencies and organizations that accredit educational programs for selected occupations. Table 2-4 diagrammatically shows the number of years of education beyond high school associated with one hundred health occupations.[4]

Needless to say, there is not enough room to describe all these fields; therefore, a small number of them has been selected for description here. We hope our readers will understand that just because this section does not describe groups such as psychiatric art therapists and marine physician assistants (serving U.S. merchant marine sailors at sea), it does not mean that these groups do not have important roles and useful tasks to perform.

2. PHYSICIANS

Physician (M.D.) Education

The educational requirements for the training of physicians was largely cast in its present mold as a result of the *Flexner Report*[5] in

---

[4] This table is taken from *Health Careers Guidebook*, United States Department of Labor, Bureau of Employment Security, (Washington, D.C.: U.S. Government Printing Office), a publication giving basic information on these occupations. Also see the annual "Guide Issue" of *Hospitals, Journal of the American Hospital Association* for a listing of approved schools for health occupations.

[5] Flexner, Abraham, *Medical Education in the United States and Canada, A Report to the Carnegie Foundation for the Advancement of Teaching*, (New York: The Carnegie Foundation, 1910).

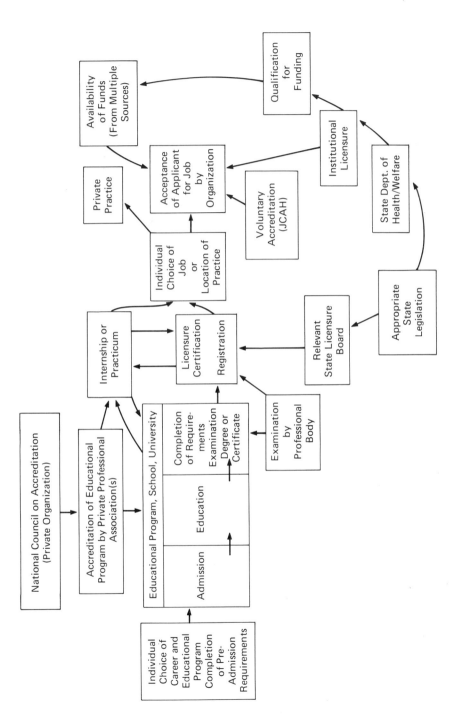

Diagram 2-1. Simplified Schematic Diagram of a Person's Entrance into a Health Profession Showing the Role of Licensure and Accreditation

Table 2-1.   List of Health Occupations

Type of Work Primary Title	Relevant and Some Alternative Titles
1. Administration	Hospital Administrator Nursing Home Administrator Clinic Manager Health Officer, Medical Care Administrator Health Planner Health Program Analyst
2. Anthropology and Sociology	Medical Anthropologist, Medical Sociologist
3. Automatic Data Processing	Computer Operator, Systems Analyst
4. Basic Sciences in the Health Field	Scientist Ecologist Anatomist Epidemiologist Biologist Microbiologist Botanist Pharmacologist Chemist
5. Biomedical Engineering	
6. Chiropractic	
7. Clinical Laboratory Service	Clinical Laboratory, Scientists, Technicians, and Technologists
8. Dentistry and Allied Services	Dentist, Dental Hygienist, Dental Assistant, Dental Laboratory Technician
9. Dietetic and Nutritional Service	Dietetic Assistant Food Service Manager Dietitian Food Service Worker Nutritionist
10. Economic Research in the Health Field	Medical Economist
11. Environmental Sanitation	Environmental Technologist Food, Milk, Sanitarian
12. Food and Drug Protective Service	Food and Drug Chemist or Microbiologist, or Inspector Health Inspector

13. Funeral Directors and Embalmers

Embalmer
Funeral Director (Mortician, Undertaker)

14. Health and Vital Statistics

Demographer
Biomathematician
Health Statistician
Vital Record Registrar

15. Health Education

Health Educator

16. Health Information and Communication

Biomedical Photographer
Medical Illustrator
Medical Writer

17. Library Services in the Health Field

Medical Librarian
Medical Library Assistant

18. Medical Records

Medical Record Administrator or Librarian or Technologist or Aide, or Technician

19. Medicine and Osteopathy

(See List of Medical Specialties)

20. Midwifery

Nurse Midwife

21. Nursing and Related Services

Registered Nurse
Licensed Practical Nurse
Home Health Aide
Attendant
Nursing Aide
Orderly

22. Occupational Therapy

Occupational Therapist
Occupational Therapy Aide
Occupational Therapy Assistant

23. Opticianry

Dispensing Optician
Optical Mechanic

24. Optometry

Optometrist
Optometric Assistant, Technician
Vision Care Aide, Technologist

(continued)

Table 2-1 continued

Type of Work Primary Title	*Relevant and Some Alternative Titles*
25. Orthotic and Prosthetic Technology	Orthotist (Orthopedic Brace Maker) Prosthetist (Prosthetic Appliance Maker)
26. Pharmacy	Pharmacist Pharmacy Aide, Assistant, Technician
27. Physical Therapy	Physical Therapist Physical Therapist Aide, Assistant
28. Podiatric Medicine	Podiatrist (Chiropodist)
29. Psychology	Psychologist (Clinical, Counseling, Developmental, School, Social)
30. Radiologic Technology	Nuclear Medicine, Radiation Therapy, Technician Radiologic Technician
31. Respiratory Therapy	Respiratory Therapist, Aide Technician (Inhalation Therapist)
32. Secretarial and Office Services	Dental, Medical Secretary, Receptionist, Office Assistant
33. Social Work	Social Worker (Caseworker), Social Work Assistant, Technician
34. Special Rehabilitation Service	Rehabilitation Specialist Music, Recreation Therapists
35. Speech Pathology and Audiology	Audiologist, Speech Pathologist
36. Veterinary Medicine	Veterinarian
37. Vocational Rehabilitation Counseling	Vocational Rehabilitation Counselor

38. Miscellaneous Health Services
   Animal Technician
   Cardiopulmonary Technician
   Community Health Aide
   Electrocardiograph Technician
   Electroencephalograph Technician
   Emergency Medical Technician
      (Ambulance Aide, Attendant, Driver)
   Extracorporeal Circulation Specialist
   Medical Assistant
   Operating Room Technician
   Ophthalmic Assistant
   Orthoptist
   Physician's Assistant
      (MEDEX, Clinical Associate,
      Community Health Medic)

Source: Health Resources Statistics, 1974. National Center for Health Statistics, U.S. Department of HEW, PHS, HSMHA (Rockville, Maryland), 1974, pp. 517–533.

Table 2-2. Estimated Number of Persons Active (Employed) in Selected
Occupations Within Each Field: 1973

Health Field and Selected Occupations	Persons Active
Total	4,403,450 to 4,448,250
Administration of Health Services	48,200
Anthropology and Sociology	1,600
Automatic Data Processing in the Health Field	4,000
Basic Sciences in the Health Field	60,000
Biomedical Engineering	11,500
Chiropractic	15,500
Clinical Laboratory Services	162,800
Dentists	105,400
Dental Hygienist	21,000
Dental Assistant	116,000
Dental Laboratory Technician	32,000
Dietetic and Nutritional Services	68,000
Economic Research in the Health Field	400
Environmental Sanitation	17,000 – 20,000
Food and Drug Protective Services	44,400
Funeral Directors and Embalmers	50,000
Health and Vital Statistics	1,350
Health Education	22,500 – 23,000
Health Information and Communication	6,700 – 9,300
Library Services in the Health Field	7,900
Medical Records	54,000
Medicine and Osteopathy	
Physician (M.D.)	333,300
Physician (D.O. Osteopathic)	12,000
Midwifery	4,200
Nursing and Related Services	
Registered Nurse	815,000
Practical Nurse	459,000
Nursing Aide, Orderly, Attendant	910,000
Home Health Aide	23,000 – 28,000
Occupational Therapy	13,200 – 14,200
Optometry and Opticianry	35,200 – 35,400
Orthotic and Prosthetic Technology	2,500 – 3,500
Pharmacy	132,900
Physical Therapy	24,600
Podiatry	7,100
Psychology	27,000
Radiologic Technology	100,000
Respiratory Therapy (Inhalation) Technician	11,000 – 12,000
Secretarial and Office Services in the Health Field	275,000 – 300,000
Social Work	33,800
Specialized Rehabilitation Services	11,050
Speech Pathology and Audiology	26,500
Veterinary Medicine	26,900
Vocational Rehabilitation Counseling	17,000
Miscellaneous	
Ambulance Attendant	207,000
Animal Technician	5,000

(continued)

Table 2-2. Estimated Number of Persons Active (Employed) in Selected Occupations Within Each Field: 1973

Health Field and Selected Occupations	Persons Active
Electrocardiograph Technician	9,500
Electroencephalograph Technician	3,500 – 4,000
Operating Room Technician	11,400
Ophthalmic Assistant	15,000 – 20,000
Orthoptist	450
Physician's Assistant	900
Surgeon's Assistant	200

Source: Health Resources Statistics, 1974. National Center for Health Statistics, U.S. Department of HEW, PHS, HSMHA (Rockville, Maryland), 1974, Table 1.

Table 2-3. Accrediting Agencies for Selected Educational Programs

Educational Program	Accrediting Agencies (Granting Approval of Educational Program)*
Blood Bank Technology	1) Council on Medical Education or the American Medical Association (AMA) 2) American Association of Blood Banks
Certified Laboratory Assistant Cytotechnology	1) Council on Medical Education or the American Medical Association (AMA) 2) American Society of Clinical Pathologists (ASCP)
Dental Hygiene	Council on Dental Education of the American Dental Association (ADA)
Dentistry	Council on Dental Education (ADA)
Dietetics	American Dietetic Association
Hospital Administration	Accrediting Commission on Graduate Education for Hospital Administration
Library Science (Special courses in hospital and medical library science)	1) American Library Association 2) Medical Library Association
Medical Assistants	1) Council on Medical Education (AMA) 2) American Association of Medical Assistants
Medical Illustration	Council on Education of the Association of Medical Illustrators
Medical Records	1) Council on Medical Education (AMA) 2) Council on Education and Registration of the American Medical Record Association
Medical Technology	1) Council on Medical Education (AMA) 2) American Society of Medical Technology
Medicine	1) Council on Medical Education (AMA) 2) Association of American Medical Colleges (AAMC)

(continued)

Table 2-3 continued

Educational Program	Accrediting Agencies (Granting Approval of Educational Program)*
Nuclear Medicine Technology	1) Council on Medical Education (AMA) 2) American College of Radiology 3) American Society of Clinical Pathologists 4) American Society of Medical Technologists 5) American Society of Radiologic Technologists 6) Society of Nuclear Medical Technologists 7) Society of Nuclear Medicine
Nurse Anesthetists	American Association of Nurse Anesthetists
Practical Nursing Professional Nursing	Approved by State Government Agencies
Occupational Therapy	1) Council on Medical Education (AMA) 2) American Occupational Therapy Association
Occupational Therapy Assistants	American Occupational Therapy Association
Operating Room Technicians	Council on Medical Education (AMA)
Osteopathy	American Osteopathic Association
Pharmacy	American Council on Pharmaceutical Education
Physical Therapy	1) Council on Medical Education (AMA) 2) American Physical Therapy Association
Podiatry	Council on Podiatry Education, American Podiatry Association
Primary Care Physician's Assistant	Council on Medical Education (AMA)
Public Health	Council on Education for Public Health
Radiation Therapy Technology Radiologic Technology	1) Council on Medical Education (AMA) 2) American College of Radiology 3) American Society of Radiologic Technologists
Respiration Therapy	1) Council on Medical Education (AMA) 2) American Association for Respiratory Therapy 3) American Thoracic Society
Social Work	Council on Social Work Education
Speech Pathology and Audiology	American Speech and Hearing Association

*Numbered agencies mean there is a joint accreditation program.
Source: Guide Issue, *Hospitals*, JAHA (Yearly). This lists names and addresses of health organizations.

Table 2–4. Calendar for Health Career Education*

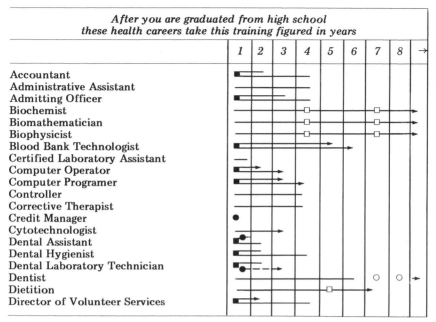

After you are graduated from high school these health careers take this training figured in years									
	1	2	3	4	5	6	7	8	→
Accountant									
Administrative Assistant									
Admitting Officer									
Biochemist									
Biomathematician									
Biophysicist									
Blood Bank Technologist									
Certified Laboratory Assistant									
Computer Operator									
Computer Programer									
Controller									
Corrective Therapist									
Credit Manager									
Cytotechnologist									
Dental Assistant									
Dental Hygienist									
Dental Laboratory Technician									
Dentist									
Dietition									
Director of Volunteer Services									

*Key to Calendar. This Calendar shows how many years of education a high school graduate should expect to spend for the representative health occupations listed here. The lines and symbols show what is customary—some people take only minimum training; many take more.

● This kind of work requires no special training beyond what you can usually get in high school.

●– – – After starting, you serve an apprenticeship or get similar organized on-the-job training.

_____ Lines and symbols used with them indicate full years. To start requires special training either in college, in a hospital or special school, or in a professional school after 1–4 years of college.

■▬▬ Special training is required, but you have a choice, each type of training taking a different number of years.

□ First symbols means you can get beginner's job after college, but will usually need more study, as well as experience, for advancement.
Graduate training ordinarily goes to or beyond master's or doctor's degree.

———→ Your planning should look beyond minimum requirements; continuing study, after entering professional practice, is important to further advancement.

○ Though the line shows the minimum to quality, more preprofessional years in college often lengthen the total training time.

(9m) Special course or on-the-job training is shown in number of months.

(continued)

Table 2-4 continued

After you are graduated from high school
these health careers take this training figured in years

	1	2	3	4	5	6	7	8	→
Educational Therapist									
Electrocardiograph Technician									
Electroencephalograph Technician									
Electronics Technician									
Executive Housekeeper									
Field Representative									
Food and Drug Inspector and Analyst									
Food Service Supervisor									
Food Service Worker									
Food Technologist									
Health Economist									
Health Information Specialist									
Health Officer									
Histologic Technician									
Home Health Aide and Homemaker									
Homemaking Rehabilitation Consultant									
Hospital Administrator									
Hospital Engineer									
Hospital Librarian									
Hospital Service Workers									
Industrial Hygienist									
Inhalation Therapist (9 m)									
Illustrators; Display Artist; Draftsman									
Laboratory Technician									
Laundry Manager									
Local Executive									
Manual Arts Therapist									
Medical Assistant									
Medical Engineering Technician									
Medical Engineer									
Medical Illustrator									
Medical Librarian									
Medical Record Librarian									
Medical Record Technician (9 m)									
Medical Secretary									
Medical Social Worker									
Medical Technologist									
Music Therapist									
Nurse, Practical (up to 18 m)									
Nurse, Professional									
Nurse Aide									
Nuclear Medical Technologist									
Nutritionist									
Occupational Therapist									
Occupational Therapy Assistant									
Office Clerical Workers									
Optician									
Optometrist									
Orderly									

(continued)

Table 2-4 continued

*After you are graduated from high school
these health careers take this training figured in years*

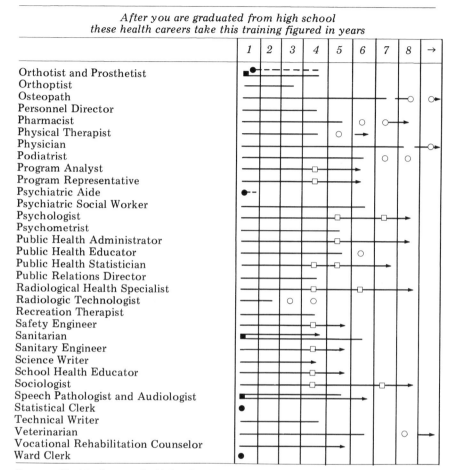

	1	2	3	4	5	6	7	8	→
Orthotist and Prosthetist									
Orthoptist									
Osteopath									
Personnel Director									
Pharmacist									
Physical Therapist									
Physician									
Podiatrist									
Program Analyst									
Program Representative									
Psychiatric Aide									
Psychiatric Social Worker									
Psychologist									
Psychometrist									
Public Health Administrator									
Public Health Educator									
Public Health Statistician									
Public Relations Director									
Radiological Health Specialist									
Radiologic Technologist									
Recreation Therapist									
Safety Engineer									
Sanitarian									
Sanitary Engineer									
Science Writer									
School Health Educator									
Sociologist									
Speech Pathologist and Audiologist									
Statistical Clerk									
Technical Writer									
Veterinarian									
Vocational Rehabilitation Counselor									
Ward Clerk									

Source: Health Careers Guidebook, U.S. Dept. of Labor, Manpower Administration (Washington, D.C.: U.S. Government Printing Office), pp. 50–51.

1910, in which Abraham Flexner criticized many of the medical schools of his day. The American Medical Association then undertook to accredit medical schools, classifying them as "A," "B," or "C," depending on their performance. Since 1938, only "A" rated medical schools have existed.

Admission to medical school requires three years of college, although four years and a B.A. degree are preponderant. Also required are a number of *pre-medical* college courses. These vary somewhat according to the medical school, but usually include biology, basic chemistry, organic chemistry, and physics. The *Medical College Admissions Test* (MCAT) is also used to evaluate the applicant's potential.

Traditionally, medical schools[6] have had four-year programs, typically divided into two years of pre-clinical or basic science courses and two years of clinical courses and practical training, the latter mostly in teaching hospitals.

A decade ago, medical school curriculums were very similar in most schools. In the interval there has developed considerable variation among the schools, including an overall trend toward increased elective time. Several schools have developed accelerated programs whereby requirements for the M.D. degree may be completed in 36 months or less.

There are 114 medical schools. Of these, six provide two years of basic medical sciences, after which students may transfer to advanced standing in a four-year school.

Medical schools are accredited by the *Liaison Committee on Medical Education*, a joint committee of the Association of American Medical Colleges and the AMA.

National Boards. The National Board examinations are standard, national examinations developed and administered by the National Board of Medical Examiners. They are given in three parts which are generally taken during the second and the final medical school years and during the internship year.

Internship and Residency Training (Graduate Medical Education). After medical school, nearly all physicians enter a year of hospital-based internship. There are two general types: *straight*, providing training in one specialty such as Internal Medicine or Surgery; and *rotating*, including more than two specialty areas.

Selection of an internship is processed by the National Intern Matching Program, which uses a computer program to match applicant and hospital preferences.

In the past, all internship programs have been approved by the A.M.A.'s Council on Medical Education. By 1975, all internships will be coordinated with residency programs and will be designated as *categorical* (straight) and *flexible*. All will be approved by the appropriate specialty bodies and the new Liaison Committee on Graduate Medical Education.

---

[6] Medical schools are either state or privately owned and, almost always, part of a university. They are represented nationally by the Association of American Medical Colleges (AAMC).

Specialization. After internship, most physicians take further specialty training in a residency program of two to five years' duration depending on the field. These programs are approved by specialty residency review committees and the Liaison Committee on Graduate Medical Education.[7] Training during this period may also include *fellowships* (usually for research or special studies). Also, most male physicians have in the past been required to serve for two years or more in the armed services (*the doctor draft*) or in the Public Health Service (See Table 2-5).

After specialty training, a physician who wishes to be certified will apply to the appropriate *specialty board.*[8] The requirments for certification by a specialty board include completion of an approved internship and residency program, written and oral examination, and varying years of practice. Completing all these requirements makes a physician *board certified* or a *diplomate* of that board.

Specialty Boards. Specialties and their specialty boards are recognized and approved by the American Board of Medical Specialties in conjunction with the AMA Council on Medical Education.

The 20 Primary Boards (Year of Incorporation) and Subspecialties or Special Certification in an Area

1. Anesthesiology (1938)
2. Colon and Rectal Surgery (1935) (Proctology)
3. Dermatology (1932)
   Dermatology and Dermatopathology
4. Family Practice (1969)
5. Internal Medicine (1936)
   Internal Medicine
   Cardiovascular Disease
   Gastroenterology
   Pulmonary Disease
   Also, certification in Endocrinology and Metabolism Hematology, Infectious Disease, Medical Oncology, Nephrology and Rheumatology

---

[7] This committee includes representatives from the American Board of Medical Specialties, American Hospital Association, American Medical Association, American Association of Medical Colleges and the Council of Medical Specialty Societies.

[8] A physician need not, however, be certified by a specialty board in order to practice a specialty.

Table 2-5.   Modal Physician's Progress*

Educational Institution	Usual Number of Years	Usual Requirements	Modal Age at Graduation
High School	12		17–18 years
College	4	Pre-Medical Courses MCAT	21–22
Medical School	4	2 Pre-Clinical Years 2 Clinical Years	25–26
Internship***	1	Completion of National Board Exams, State Licensure	26–27
Residency	2–5+	May also include fellowship	28–32+
Military Service**	2	May include internship and/or residency or come prior to residency	30–34+
Specialty Requirements			
Specialty Practice (Research, Teaching, Administrative, etc.)	—	Examinations, Experience and Others	
General Practice and other careers			

Graduate of Foreign Medical Schools

ECFMG Exam

*See American Medical Association, *Directory of Approved Internships and Residencies, 1971–1972.* The Association, Chicago, Illinois, p. 9.

**No Longer Required.

***In some cases, internship is now not required. The graduate goes directly into a residency program.

6. Neurological Surgery (1940) (Neurosurgery)
7. Obstetrics and Gynecology (1930)
    Obstetrics and Gynecology, Gynecologic Oncology, Maternal and Fetal Medicine, Reproductive Endocrinology
8. Ophthalmology (1917)
9. Orthopedic Surgery (1934)
10. Otolaryngology (1924)
    Otolaryngology
    Limited Branches
11. Pathology (1936)
    Singly or in various combinations: anatomic, clinical, forensic, chemical and radioisotopic pathology, hematology, neuropathology, medical microbiology, blood banking, and dermatopathology
12. Pediatrics (1933)
    Pediatrics
    Pediatric Cardiology
    Pediatric Hematology-Oncology
    Pediatric Nephrology
    Neonatal-Perinatal Medicine
13. Physical Medicine and Rehabilitation (1947)
14. Plastic Surgery (1939)
15. Preventive Medicine (1948)
    General Preventive Medicine
    Aerospace Medicine
    Occupational Medicine
    Public Health
16. Psychiatry and Neurology (1934)
    Psychiatry
    Neurology
    Psychiatry and Neurology
    Child Psychiatry
    Neurology with special competence in child neurology
17. Radiology (1934)
    Diagnostic Radiology
    Therapeutic Radiology
    Nuclear Radiology
    Radiological Physics
    Therapeutic Radiological Physics
    Diagnostic Radiological Physics
    Medical Nuclear Physics
18. Surgery (1937) (General Surgery)
    Surgery, Pediatric Surgery

19. Thoracic Surgery (1948)
20. Urology (1935)

There are also two *conjoint boards* based on cooperation of two or more primary boards:[9]

1. *Nuclear Medicine*, a conjoint board of Internal Medicine, Pathology and Radiology. (1971)
2. *Allergy and Immunology*, a conjoint board of Internal Medicine and Pediatrics. (1971)

Physician Licensure.   Medical licensure is on a state-by-state basis. If a physician is licensed in one state, it does not allow him to practice medicine in another state without obtaining its license. (Special temporary state licenses are granted to resident physicians working in hospitals.)

In all states, the requirements, which are set forth in Medical Practice Acts, include passing an examination. Traditionally, these have been developed and administered by state boards. In many states, certification by the National Board of Medical Examiners is accepted in lieu of state examinations.

In recent years, there has been wide acceptance by the states of the Federation Licensing Examination (FLEX),[10] developed by the Federation of Licensing Boards.

Many states recognize, in lieu of examination, licenses granted by certain other states (reciprocity).

Foreign Medical Graduates.   (FMG) Graduates of foreign medical schools (except Canadian) who wish to take an approved U.S. internship or residency must pass an examination prepared by the Educational Council for Foreign Medical Graduates (ECFMG).[11]

Osteopathic Physicians (D.O.)

Physicians (M.D.) and *Osteopathic Physicians (D.O.)* are often grouped together because their education and mode of practice are quite

---

[9] *Dictionary of Medical Specialists.* Various Editions. Marquis, Who's Who. Chicago.

[10] John P. Hubbard, "Evaluation, Certification and Licensure in Medicine," *JAMA* 225, 4 (July 23, 1973): 401.

[11] The Council is sponsored by the American Hospital Association, the American Medical Association, the Association of American Medical Colleges, the Association for Hospital and Medical Education and the Federation of State Medical Boards.

similar. Until recently, *osteopathy* and *medicine* have constituted separate professions with separate education and hospitals. Recently there has been more interchange between the two.

Osteopathy originated as a reform movement in American medicine, originally propounded in 1874 by Dr. Andrew Taylor Still. Today there are seven colleges of osteopathy accredited by the American Osteopathic Association, whose graduates receive the degree of Doctor of Osteopathy (D.O.).

The content of osteopathic education is the same as that in M.D. medical schools except that osteopaths have additional class hours devoted to osteopathic manipulation.

Over time, differences in approaches to treatment between medicine and osteopathy have narrowed to the point where, in California, these two professions have completely merged.

Osteopathy has been defined (1956) as "a system of medical practice based on the theory that disease is due chiefly to mechanical derangement in tissues, placing emphasis on restoration of structural integrity by manipulation of the parts. The uses of medicines, surgery, proper diet, psychotherapy, and other measures are included in osteopathy."

In 1963, about half of the 12,000 practicing osteopaths were located in Michigan, Missouri, Ohio, Pennsylvania, and Texas (excluding California, where M.D.'s and D.O.'s have merged). In recent years, over 70 percent of the students entering osteopathic colleges have a bachelor's degree. One year of internship after the D.O. degree is customary, and beyond that there is further training leading to membership in one of twelve osteopathic specialty boards. While most M.D.'s specialize, most D.O.'s practice family medicine. Licensure is required for practice. Nearly all states grant osteopathic physicians the same practice privileges as medical physicians, although a few states restrict osteopathic use of drugs and surgery.

Table 2-6 shows the number of medical and osteopathic physicians in various specialties.

The word "medicine" is used in three ways. One is to refer to all activities of physicians (as in "the practice of medicine"). The second use is in distinction to "surgery" (as in "internal medicine"). The third use is to distinguish medicine from osteopathy. Sometimes osteopathic physicians refer to M.D.'s as allopathic physicians.*

---

*Dorland's *Medical Dictionary* (23[d] Edition), says: Allopathy is "an erroneous designation for the regular system of medicine and surgery".

Table 2-6.   Type of Practice and Primary Specialty of Active Physicians: United States, 1973

	Active M.D.s (Dec. 31, 1973)					
	Total[1]		Patient care			Other profes-sional activity[2]
			Office-based practice	Hospital-based practice		
Primary specialty	Number	Percent		Training programs	Full-time physician staff	
Total	324,367	100.0	201,435	58,252	35,570	29,110
Percent	100.0	—	62.1	18.0	11.0	9.0
General practice[3]	69,823	21.5	51,220	8,504	5,335	4,764
Specialty practice	254,544	78.5	150,215	49,748	30,235	24,346
Medical specialties	86,924	26.8	48,689	19,333	9,576	9,326
Allergy	1,640	0.5	1,418	—	76	146
Cardiovascular diseases	6,159	1.9	4,345	—	815	999
Dermatology	4,340	1.3	3,188	623	268	261
Gastroenterology	1,983	0.6	1,348	—	257	378
Internal medicine	49,899	15.4	25,315	14,163	5,328	5,093
Pediatrics[4]	20,849	6.4	12,135	4,547	2,182	1,985
Pulmonary diseases	2,054	0.6	940	—	650	464
Surgical specialties	103,745	32.0	71,700	19,428	8,369	4,248
Anesthesiology	12,196	3.8	8,217	1,820	1,410	749
Colon and rectal surgery	658	0.2	602	27	15	14
General surgery	30,857	9.5	19,040	7,885	2,740	1,192
Neurological surgery	2,809	0.9	1,851	586	221	151
Obstetrics and gynecology	20,494	6.3	14,823	3,311	1,396	964
Ophthalmology	10,496	3.2	8,208	1,448	502	338
Orthopedic surgery	10,587	3.5	7,450	1,970	875	292
Otolaryngology	5,484	1.7	4,068	827	403	186
Plastic surgery	1,991	0.6	1,497	303	118	73

Thoracic surgery	1,875	0.6	1,283	264	213	115
Urology	6,298	1.9	4,661	987	476	174
Psychiatry and neurology	28,804	8.9	14,387	4,944	5,581	3,892
Child psychiatry	2,362	0.7	1,293	322	329	418
Neurology	3,741	1.2	1,614	941	542	644
Psychiatry	22,701	7.0	11,480	3,681	4,710	2,830
Other specialties	35,071	10.8	15,439	6,043	6,709	6,880
Aerospace medicine	779	0.2	220	43	173	343
General preventive medicine	769	0.2	212	50	51	456
Occupational medicine	2,374	0.7	1,639	7	73	655
Pathology[5]	11,498	3.5	3,782	2,638	2,811	2,267
Physical medicine and rehabilitation	1,569	0.5	554	286	572	157
Public health	2,737	0.8	531	40	151	2,015
Radiology[6]	15,345	4.7	8,501	2,979	2,878	987

1. Excludes 5,644 M.D.s with addresses unknown, 13,744 unclassified M.D.s, and an estimated 12,000 doctors of osteopathy, for whom recent data are not available.
2. Includes medical teaching, administration, research, and other.
3. Includes no specialty reported and other specialties not listed.
4. Includes pediatric allergy and pediatric cardiology.
5. Includes forensic pathology.
6. Includes diagnostic radiology and therapeutic radiology.

Source: AMA Center for Health Services Research and Development: Distribution of Physicians in the United States, 1973. Regional, State, County, Metropolitan Areas. G.A. Roback, Chicago, American Medical Association, 1974.

References

American Medical Association, *Directory of Approved Internships and Residencies* (Chicago: The Association, Yearly).

Association of American Medical Colleges, *Medical School Admissions Requirements* (Washington, D.C.: The Association, Yearly).

Advisory Board for Medical Specialists, Inc., *The Directory of Medical Specialists*, Fifteenth Edition (Chicago: Marquis-Who's Who, periodically).

"Medical Education in the United States," *Journal of the American Medical Association*, November, Yearly.

Rosemary Stevens, *American Medicine and the Public Interest* (New Haven: Yale University Press, 1971). A study of the evolution of medical specialization in the United States.

3. DENTISTS

A minimum of two years of college is required for admission to dental school. About 50 percent of dental students have a bachelor's degree, and this percentage is increasing. Most dental schools require four academic years to obtain the D.M.D. (Doctor of Dental Medicine) or D.D.S. (Doctor of Dental Surgery) degree, although some now have a three calendar year program. For all practical purposes, there is no difference in the D.M.D. and D.D.S. degrees. Dentists and Physicians are both Doctors, so it is inappropriate to say "Dentists and Doctors."

To be admitted to dental school it is necessary to take the Dental Aptitude Test (DAT) prepared by the Division of Educational Measurements of the American Dental Association (ADA). In the first two years (basic science years) of dental school, in some universities, the dental students take the same courses as the medical students, with the addition of oral anatomy, oral pathology, and other pre-clinical dental science courses. The third and fourth years are usually the clinical years, when students treat patients under faculty supervision in the school's clinics or community facilities. Now some schools are blending the basic sciences and clinical years. Dental internships and residencies are not required for general practice, but are required for board certification in a dental specialty. The eight recognized dental specialties are:

1. *Endodontics* (root treatment).
2. *Oral Pathology* (the study of diseased oral tissues).

3. *Oral Surgery*
4. *Orthodontics* (straightening of the teeth).
5. *Pedodontics* (children's dentistry).
6. *Periodontology* or *Periodontics* (treatment of the gums, bone, and other tissues surrounding the teeth).
7. *Prosthodontics* (replacing missing teeth).
8. *Public Health Dentistry*

In addition to the dental degree, all states and the District of Columbia require a written and practical examination for licensure. A certificate from the National Board of Dental Examiners is accepted in place of the written exam in all states except Delaware and Arizona.[12] Regional Dental Examining Boards have been established and successful completion of those examinations is accepted as satisfying the practical examination requirement for several specified states.

Canadian dental education is accepted in most states, but graduates from other foreign dental schools must take additional training in a U.S. Dental School before being examined for licensure. The Science Achievement Examination for Dentistry allows up to 2 years advance placement in a U.S. Dental School. The foreign graduate must take the last two clinical years in a U.S. Dental School.

About 90 percent of active dentists are in private practice and most are in general practice, although specialization is increasing. Other careers include research, teaching, and administration. There is a growing interest in allied dental occupations including:

- *Dental Hygienist*—requires two years of formal education and training as well as state licensure.
- *Dental Assistant*—assist the dentist in patient care (no educational requirements although there are many dental assistant training programs of one or more years' duration. National examination and certification is possible).
- *Dental Laboratory Technicians*—(sometimes called Denturists in Canada) who perform certain mechanical and technical procedures involved in the fabrication of artificial teeth and dentures.

Emerging programs train *Dental Therapists, Expanded Duty Auxiliaries*, or *Expanded Duty Dental Assistants* (EDDAs). This development is similar in concept to Physician's Assistants. These new personnel undertake a wider range of tasks than dental hygienists, but

[12] *Manpower Supply and Educational Statistics for Dentists and Dental Auxiliaries*, U.S. Dept. of HEW, Public Health Service, Bethesda, Md. (April 1972), p. 1.

a smaller range than dentists. Dental schools are now providing courses for dentists in Dental Auxiliary Utilization (DAU) and Training in Expanded Auxiliary Management (TEAM).

4. NURSES

The following is a brief description of nursing, particularly nursing education, which is designed to provide a basic background for the many current issues and changes in the field, and its relation to other health professions.

Professional Nurses

Professional nurses are generally known in the United States as registered nurses (RNs). (In the past the terms *graduate* and *trained nurse* have also been used.)

Education. There are three basic types of educational programs which prepare registered nurses: diploma, baccalaureate, and associate degree.

Diploma programs. These are typically three-year programs in hospital-based schools of nursing. These schools had their origin in the training schools for nursing which began to be established in the 1870s and which were originally based on the nursing education principles newly established in London by Florence Nightingale.[13]

Until recently, the great majority of nursing graduates came from diploma schools. With the increasing development of college programs, the percentage of diploma graduates has declined and the total number of such programs is diminishing.[14]

Baccalaureate programs. These are four-or five-year college or

---

[13] The first three of these schools were the Bellevue Training School for Nurses, the Connecticut Training School (New Haven) and Massachusetts General Hospital Training School (all established in 1873).

Significant for the future development of nursing education in the United States was the fact that most of these schools were developed as integral parts of hospitals and became closely associated with the provision of hospital nursing services in an essentially apprentice system.

[14] Contributing to the decline in the hospital programs has been the increased costs associated with improved curriculums and decreased emphasis on meeting hospital service needs.

university-based programs which lead to the Bachelor of Science degree. Clinical experience is obtained in university or affiliated teaching hospitals.

The first school established within a university was at the University of Minnesota (1910). Such schools began to come to prominence in the 1930s and have steadily expanded in numbers; in 1969–70 they graduated 21 percent of new nurses.

Associate degree programs.   These are two-year programs, usually based in junior and community colleges, leading to an Associate in Arts degree. Practical experience is obtained in affiliated hospitals. Such programs were first established in 1952[15] and have rapidly increased, graduating 27 percent of new nurses in 1969-70.

Nursing educational programs are approved by state agencies, such as the state education department or nursing board. In addition, a voluntary *accreditation program* is carried out by the National League for Nursing and most schools and programs are so accredited.

Licensure.   The first licensure acts for nurses were passed in 1903, and by 1923 all states and the District of Columbia had such laws. These statutes, usually called *nursing practice acts* are administered by nursing boards.[16]

In a few states, licensure is not mandatory for the practice of nursing; their licensure laws merely prohibiting unlicensed persons from using the title "registered nurse;" i.e., these laws are voluntary, protecting the title, but not regulating nursing practice. Licensure examinations, required in all states, are administered by the nursing boards, from an examination pool maintained by the National League of Nursing.

Advanced Training and Specialization.   There are many *master's degree* programs which have been developed for the advanced training of nurses in nursing education, administration, and clinical specialties.[17]

---

[15] By seven colleges in cooperation with the Cooperative Research Project in Junior and Community College Education, Teachers College, Columbia University.

[16] Variously named Board of Nursing, Board of Nursing Examiners, Board of Nursing Education and Nurse Registration, etc.

[17] Advanced education for professional nurses had its origins in programs established at Teachers College, Columbia University: a course for those who would be teaching in nursing schools (1900) and courses in public health nursing (1910).

The clinical specialty programs include public health (community health), medical-surgical nursing, maternal and child health, mental health, rehabilitation, and cardiovascular nursing.

A number of *doctoral degree* programs in nursing have been established since the mid-1940s. This level of education is being encouraged by many nursing educators for nurses pursuing teaching and research careers in collegiate programs.

"Nurse-clinicians, clinical nursing specialists." The increasing popularity of educational programs in the clinical specialties is a manifestation of a trend toward making available opportunities for professional advancement for nurses by increasing clinical skills as opposed to the traditional routes of teaching or administration.[18] Other examples of the development of special clinical skills are the hospital in-service training programs for nurses in intensive care and coronary care units; and the *nurse practitioner* programs which have been developed in ambulatory care settings (see Chapter 6).

A related development has been the trend toward relieving nurses of non-nursing administrative and clerical tasks in order that more of their energy can be devoted to patient care. One manifestation of this trend has been the establishment of *ward manager*, (unit manager) positions in many hospitals.

Two older types of nurse specialists are particularly noteworthy: *nurse midwives* and *nurse anesthetists*.

Nurse Anesthetists. Nurse anesthetists have been employed in hospital surgical units since before 1900 and the first school for the formal training of nurses in the administration of anesthesia was established at Lakeside Hospital in Cleveland about 1910. Programs now are generally of 18-months' duration and lead to certification.

Nurse Midwives.[19] Nurse midwives are registered nurses with special training in prenatal and postpartum care and the management of normal labor and delivery.

The first U.S. training school was established in New York City in 1932. Nurse midwives trained in Britain had been practicing with the

[18] For example, the usual route for advancement in hospital nursing has been from staff nurse to head nurse, nursing supervisor, assistant director, and, ultimately, director of nurses.

[19] Lay midwives, often called "granny midwives," have for many years practiced among poor populations, especially in the rural south. They are licensed in many states, although in many instances no new licenses are being issued.

Frontier Nursing Service in Kentucky since 1927, and a School of Midwifery was established there in 1939.

Programs, leading to certification, are from 8–24 months, the latter leading to a master's degree.

Practical Nurses

Practical nurses are recognized in all states as *licensed* practical nurses (LPN) or as licensed *vocational* nurses (LVN) (California and Texas).

The first educational programs in practical nursing were established under provisions of the Vocational Education Act of 1917 (Smith-Hughes Act). They are based in vocational and technical schools, hospitals and community colleges and are generally of eight to fifteen months' duration.

The licensing agency in most states is the state nursing board; there is a separate board of practical nursing examiners in several states. In about half the states, the law is compulsory, regulating practice; in the others, it is voluntary, protecting the title.[20]

Nursing Aides (Nursing Assistants)

Nursing aides are important personnel in hospitals and nursing homes. They perform many tasks related to personal care of patients. Educational requirements are those specified by the hiring institution, usually some years of high school. Training is on the job with scope, duration and formality varying greatly among institutions.

Associations

American Nurses' Association (ANA). This is the professional association for registered nurses and is particularly concerned with nursing practice and the nursing profession.

National League for Nursing (NLN). This association includes registered and practical nurses, nursing aides, and other (non-nursing) persons interested in nursing. It is particularly concerned with the improvement of organized nursing services and educational programs.

American College of Nurse Midwives. This is the professional association for nurse midwives. Its activities include the accreditation of training programs and the certification of their graduates.

[20] The term "waivered" practical nurse refers to those who, in certain states, have been licensed on the basis of previous practice, without the educational requirements.

American Association of Nurse Anesthetists. This is the professional association for nurse anesthetists. The requirements for membership include a qualifying examination.

The National Federation of Licensed Practical Nurses is the professional association for practical nurses.

References

Mary M. Roberts, *American Nursing—History and Interpretation* (New York: The Macmillan Company, 1954).

Facts About Nursing: A Statistical Summary (New York: The American Nurses Association). Annually or Biannually.

Nursing and Nursing Education in the United States, Report of the Committee for the Study of Nursing Education and Report of a Survey by Josephine Goldmark (New York: The Macmillan Company, 1923).

Esther Lucille Brown, *Nursing for the Future* (New York: Russell Sage Foundation, 1948).

National Commission for the Study of Nursing and Nursing Education, *An Abstract for Action* (New York: McGraw-Hill Company, 1970).

5. A SAMPLING OF OTHER HEALTH PROFESSIONS

Herein are a few short descriptions of a sampling of health occupations chosen to show the range and variation that exists. The number of different health occupations is steadily growing. Space does not permit inclusion of all of them.

Administration (Health Administration, Hospital Administration, Health Management, etc.). Educational programs in health services administration are located in medical schools, schools of public health, business schools, and schools of government or public administration, or in a combination of the above. Courses and degrees are provided at the baccalaureate, master, and doctorate levels. The Association of University Programs in Health Administration (AUPHA) is a voluntary organization which represents most of these programs.

Dieticians and Nutritionists. Dieticians specialize in feeding people, and their profession is largely hospital based. They can specialize in teaching, research, administration, and therapy (planning special menus and diets). The nutritionist is, in practice, an educator who often works in a public health setting. Both professions require a college education. Master and doctorate degrees are available. Dieticians ordinarily take a one-year internship, and post-college education is recommended for nutritionists. The American Dietetic Association (ADA) serves as the professional association for both groups. The dietician brings knowledge of, and skills in, nutrition and/or management to the feeding of individuals and groups. The nutritionist is concerned with carrying out nutritional programs for the promotion of health and prevention of disease, consults with other professionals, and provides education for both health professionals and the public.

Medical Record Librarians. This is primarily a hospital occupation. There are three routes to this career: (a) by experience without formal education, (b) by a twelve-month hospital certificate school which admits students with a minimum of two years of study in college, and (c) by four-year college programs which award a bachelor's degree of medical record administration or medical record science. Graduates of the four-year program are eligible to take the examination to qualify as a registered record librarian (RRL). *Medical Record Technicians* require from nine to twelve months after high school.

Medical Technology and Related Services

Medical Technologist. A registered medical technologist requires three years of college and one year in one of about 800 approved training schools. Afterwards, passing the examination confers the title M.T. (ASCP). This ASCP stands for the American Society for Clinical Pathologists, which helps administer the exam.

Cytotechnologist. Two years of college, six months in an approved school, and six months' experience in an acceptable laboratory are required. After this, passing the certifying exam allows one to use the designation C.T. (ASCP).

Blood Bank Technologists. These are registered medical technologists who have had an additional year's training in a blood bank school approved by the American Association of Blood Banks. The examination confers the title M.T. (ASCP) B.B.

Histologic Technicians. These require a year of supervised training in a clinical pathology laboratory, beyond high school. Examination confers certification as H.T. (ASCP).

Nuclear Medical Technology. For people with an M.T. (ASCP) or a B.S. degree in biologic or chemical sciences, plus a year's training.

Certified Laboratory Assistants. These work under the supervision of medical technologists and pathologists. It requires one year of hospital training beyond high school, and passing an examination confers the letters CLA.

Electrocardiograph (ECG or EKG) Technicians and *Electroencephalograph (EEG) Technicians.* These are trained on the job and usually require a high school education.

Occupational Therapy requires four years of college leading to a bachelor of science in occupational therapy. About thirty college and universities are approved for these programs. In addition, nine to ten months of clinical training is required. There is also an optional additional eighteen months of academic and clinical training for advanced standing, and some master's degree programs. Passing the national registration exam confers the degree O.T.R. *Occupational Therapy Assistants* require high school graduation plus a training program. Orthopedic and Prosthetic Appliance Makers make and fit artificial limbs. The *prosthetist* makes and fits artificial limbs and the *orthotist* makes and fits orthopedic braces, both working from a physician's prescription.

Eye Care. *Opthalmology* is a specialty in medicine. An *optician* dispenses eyeglasses prescribed by a physician. He fits and grinds glasses and contact lenses. Grinding is also done by optical wholesalers and by *optical technicians.* There are several schools of optical technology. Opticians are high school graduates who have had four to five years' apprenticeship. A few states license these two occupations. An *optometrist* has the degree Doctor of Optometry (O.D.) and is licensed to examine eyes for vision problems, disease, and other abnormalities. He prescribes and fits glasses. The American Optometric Association estimates that optometrists perform 75 percent of all eye examinations. Training requires two years of college and three to four years in a college of optometry. All states license optometrists, which requires an examination. An *orthoptist* helps people with crossed eyes, using instruction and exercises, and works under the guidance of an ophthalmologist. A college degree is required, plus a year in school or training. The American Orthoptic Council gives an examination and certification.

Pharmacy is an applied physical science: the practice of preparing, preserving, and dispensing drugs and medicines. For many pharmacists it combines a professional and business career. About 80 percent of all pharmacists are in retail or community pharmacy. (See Chapter 9). Some of these drug stores limit themselves to health products, while others sell a wide range of products. About 10 percent of pharmacists work in hospital-based pharmacies. The remainder works in industry, government, or teaching.

Pharmacy requires five years of education after high school for a B.S. in Pharmacy. Prior to 1960, four years were required. Of the current five years, the first two are pre-professional and the last three are professional. Transfer students are accepted after the first (one-four) and second (two-three) years from junior colleges or liberal arts schools. The three professional years include the study of pharmaceutical chemistry, pharmacognosy (the study of natural drugs from plants and animals), pharmacology (the action of drugs in the body), toxicology (the effects of poisons on the body, and antidotes), pharmacy administration, and clinical pharmacy. There are 73 pharmacy schools in the U.S. accredited by the American Council of Pharmaceutical Education. Master and doctorate degrees of pharmacy are also awarded. Licensure ordinarily requires a degree from an accredited school; an apprenticeship or internship of six months to one year under the supervision of a licensed pharmacist; and passage of the state board examination.

Physical Therapy qualifications can be obtained in three ways: (a) a four-year bachelor's degree program, (b) a twelve-month certificate course for people with a bachelor's degree, and (c) master's degree training. Physical Therapists are licensed.

Podiatry. *Podiatrists* or *Chiropodists* (these terms are synonymous) diagnose and treat diseases and deformities of the feet. There are five accredited schools of podiatry requiring two years of college before admission, and four years before receiving the DSC (Doctor of Surgical Chiropody) or Pod.D. (Doctor of Podiatry) degree. Internship is optional and not required for state licensure, although examination is. All states license podiatrists.

Public Health includes a variety of specialized professional careers. Schools of public health are university-based and provide graduate education to a wide range of health personnel on the delivery of health services to large populations (in contrast to providing care to individual patients). Some major areas of education and research include:

Environmental Health (air pollution control, accident prevention, occupational medicine, industrial safety, control of radiological
   hazards, sewage and solid waste disposal, sanitation engineering,
   provision of clean water supplies, and fluoridation)
Population Studies (family planning, population control)
Demography (the study of population size, distribution, and charac-
   teristics)
Biostatistics (the application of statistics to health problems)
Nutrition (the relationship between food use and production and
   health)
Infectious Diseases and Tropical Public Health
Epidemiology (the study of the impact of disease on populations)
Maternal and Child Health
Public Health Nursing
Public Health Dentistry
Health Services Administration (medical care administration)

Radiology. Radiologic Technologists (also called *X-Ray Technicians*) assist the radiologist. Various forms of training are possible,
including a 24-month program in an approved hospital-based school.
Some of these programs extend over a four-year period and entitle
the graduate to the degree of Bachelor of Science in X-Ray Technology. The hospital schools usually charge no tuition and have two
to six students, on average.

Social Work. Professional social workers have two years of graduate education leading to the Master of Social Work (MSW) degree in
an accredited school of social work. The curriculum combines class-
room instruction and field experience covering social welfare policy
and services, human behavior and social environment and social work
practice. Areas of concentration include service to individuals (social
case work) groups (social group work) and communities (community
organization), administration, research, and social policy. Social
workers practice both inside the health field and in other areas. Major
practice settings include health, mental health, child welfare, family
services, aging, juvenile, and adult justice, community service and
planning.

There are also accredited four-year bachelor's degree programs
whose graduates are usually called social work assistants or aides.

Neighborhood Aides have a high school education or less. A major qualification is familiarity with the living conditions and values of the population being served and, they often function as liaison personnel between clients and social work staff.

Veterinary Medicine (care of animals). Veterinarians receive the D.V.M. (or V.M.D.) degree. Veterinarians are largely in private practice. They take care of pets and other animals, such as race horses and breeding stock, which can be very valuable to their owners, who insist on excellent care to protect their investments. The work of veterinarians affects human health because veterinarians are involved in research on animals which has application to human medicine. There are diseases which are transmitted from animals to man, and the health of cattle, sheep, and other animals is important because these animals are sources of human food.

Other Practitioners or Sectarian Practitioners. The American Medical Association refers to such practitioners as "cultists" and "quacks" because it is believed they do not accept the principles of modern scientific medicine. They have little or no contact with the "regular" medical occupations. According to the AMA, it is unethical for physicians to have any dealing with these practitioners. Needless to say, these practitioners view their roles and skills as having an important and useful function.

Chiropractic is a system of mechanical therapeutics based on the principle that the nervous system largely determines the state of health. Treatment consists primarily of chiropractic manipulation usually of the spinal column. Some chiropractors ("mixers" as opposed to "straights"), also use physiotherapy and dietary modification and radiology for diagnosis. Drugs and Surgery are not used. There are about 20,000 licensed chiropractors mostly in California (20%), New York, Texas, Missouri, and Pennsylvania. Licensure usually requires the completion of two years of college, and then a four-year chiropractic course in one of ten approved schools, leading to the degree of doctor of chiropractic (D.C.).

Naprapaths rely on water baths and steam for therapy.

Naturopaths rely on special foods and diets.

Folk Medicine refers to home remedies based on cultural tradition, rather than on scientific evidence; e.g., the expression "an apple a day keeps the doctor away," or the practice of always wearing a copper bracelet to stay healthy.

Faith Healers use the power of religious faith to cure illness.[21] For example, *Christian Science* does not accept the idea that medicine can cure illness; only the Deity can. There are Christian Science Practitioners and Nurses who provide spiritual help, advice, and physical assistance to the ill.

Reference

Job Descriptions and Organizational Analysis for Hospitals and Related Health Services, Revised Edition (Washington, D.C.: U.S. Government Printing Office, 1971).

[21] The Indian Health Service has encouraged some use of Navaho native faith healers are intermediaries between the Navaho Indians and modern medicine, in order to maintain Navaho tribal customs and the psychological benefits of their healing ceremonies.

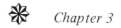

Chapter 3

Paying for Care

1. INTRODUCTION

There are several basic ways that health services are paid for and provided. They each have different characteristics and problems associated with them.

Direct, Out-of-Pocket Payment. Here the individual patient comes to an agreement (contracts) directly with the provider (doctor, hospital, etc.). Those patients who cannot pay all their bill receive care for free or less than the usual price as a form of *charity*. This was either through private donations to hospitals, etc., for care of the poor or by individual doctors through the use of a *sliding scale* of fees, whereby the wealthy would pay more in order to support the care of the poor. Prior to the extensive growth of health insurance from the 1940s to the present, this was the customary way in which health care was paid for. Direct payment is still customary for low cost health care items.

Provision of Service. The army health service, city hospitals, Indian Health Service, and the V.A. all receive an annual budget and in return provide a fixed amount of service (so many hospital beds, clinics, doctors, etc.). The amount of services provided may be more or less adequate. The recipient of care pays nothing directly and perhaps nothing indirectly through taxes. For this reason, this form of service payment is frequently used to provide health care for the poor. It relies largely on the individual doctors employed by the service to decide who is to receive care among eligible population and how much care they receive, based on the doctors' definition of medical need.[1]

Insurance and Prepayment. Individuals make a contractual agreement, either singly or in groups, with an insurer who promises to pay for an agreed-upon range of services under specified conditions. The insurer can pay money directly to the subscriber, or to the provider of services (e.g., Blue Cross, Blue Shield). One device to promote widespread coverage of moderate and high income families is the use of *community rating*, whereby all people in the same area (e.g., state) pay the same monthly premium. Another way to do this is to subsidize premium payments for the poor. A third way is government health insurance (Medicare and Medicaid). This form of payment requires careful specification of risks to be covered so that the insurer can estimate the probable size of his benefit payments. It also is subject to such problems as overutilization of services. If a self-pay patient uses a great many health services, it is his concern. If other members of an insured group use a great many services, it increases each member's premium payments and, therefore, each member is affected by the behavior of others (a phenomenon economists call *externalities*). In contrast, the direct provision of services has a more controllable and predictable budgeted level of expenditure.

The difference between prepayment and insurance: Several different definitions are in use:*

1. Blue Cross, Blue Shield, and prepaid group practices (e.g., Kaiser-Permanente, HMOs) are *prepayment plans.* They either contract with providers of service or provide the service themselves (HMOs). In contrast, insurance companies do not contract with providers, but only with subscribers, and rather than providing care, they are said to provide *insurance.* Medicare is separately classified.
2. *Prepayment* is payment in advance for services to be used. An expectant mother may pay her doctor in advance for delivering her baby. There may be no pooling of risk in this case. By this

---

[1] This is not the same as service benefits, as provided by Blue Cross, Blue Shield, and prepaid groups.

*The historical reason for these differences lie, in part, with the competition between Blue Cross, Blue Shield and Insurance Companies. Blue Cross Enabling Legislation was put forward with the argument of their uniqueness summed up in the word "prepayment". Sometimes, Insurance Companies have argued that these State laws provide unfair competitive advantages to BC-BS. They argue that BC-BS provides insurance and should be viewed in the same fashion as Insurance Companies.

definition, Blue Cross and the insurance companies provide *insurance*. Perhaps Medicare Part A, under this definition, would be, in part, prepayment because the worker pays money for Social Security before he becomes 65 and eligible for benefits.

3. There is no difference between prepayment and insurance. By this definition, Blue Cross and Blue Shield are nonprofit insurance companies.

4. Other special definitions of prepayment include combinations of the following features: service benefits, contract with providers, agreement on charges to subscribers, nonprofit, *first dollar coverage*, coverage of a large proportion of the subscribers' health care costs (comprehensive benefits), etc. This definition is, in effect, similar to (1) since Blue Cross and Kaiser both fit these characteristics and insurance companies do not.

Of these different definitions, (1) and (4) are most frequently used.

Prepayment Plans, HMOs, Kaiser-Permanente, etc. These plans combine the provision of service with fixed monthly payments by subscribers and the pooling of risk. They are a combination of II and III, described above.

Charitable Contributions, Endowment Funds, Revenue from Other Miscellaneous Sources Used to Provide Care.

Payment of Physicians

Fee for Service. A fee is charged the patient for each task or *procedure* performed; with differing fees according to the length and difficulty of the task performed.

Sliding Fee Scale. Variation in the fee charged, according to the patient's income. The poor paying less and the rich paying more for the same service.

Relative Value Scale. A listing of procedures performed. Each procedure is given an index number which reflects the relative length and complexity of the task. This index number is then multiplied by a dollar amount to obtain the appropriate fee. The California Relative Value Scale is best known.

Usual and Customary Fee. The fee for a given procedure that is usually charged by the doctor and other doctors in the area.

Capitation. A fixed amount of money for a given time period is given to the practitioner for each patient under his/her care, regardless of the amount of care that patient receives. Those patients who sign up with the practitioner to pay for care by capitation constitute that practitioner's *panel* of patients.

Closed panel practice means that the practitioner will only care for patients on his panel. This term has been applied to the prepaid group practices and HMO's.

Salary. A fixed payment, regardless of the amount of work performed or the number of patients seen.

Other Payment Methods. Physicians working in group practices or in hospitals are paid in a variety of ways that can be very complex mixes of salary, fee for service, percentages of revenue generated, etc.

Free Services. Practitioners may not charge for care provided. Sometimes a physician on a hospital staff may provide an agreed-upon amount of service in the hospital without pay, in exchange for his hospital admitting privileges.

2. HEALTH INSURANCE AND PREPAYMENT

Definition of Insurance and Health Insurance

Insurance can be defined as "protection by written contract against the hazards (in whole or in part) of the happenings of specified fortuitous events."[2]

Health Insurance can be defined as "protection against the costs of hospital and medical care of lost income arising from an illness or injury."

Characteristics of Health Insurance Policies

coverage—types of illness, types of treatment for which the policy holder will be recompensed (covered)

age limits—both for new applicants and renewals

exclusions—"specified hazards for which a policy will not provide benefit payments"

benefits—amount of money to be paid for type of illness or treatment

policy term—time period covered by the policy

[2] Quotations from Health Insurance Institute *Source Book of Health Insurance Data* New York, Yearly.

preexisting conditions—physical conditions of the insured person which existed prior to the issuance of his policy which may or may not be covered

grace period—"a specified time after a policy's premium payment is due in which the protection of the policy continues subject to actual receipt of premium within that time"

rider—an amendment to the policy expanding or decreasing benefits

time limits—the period of time in which notice of claim or proof of loss must be filed in order to obtain benefits

upper limits of coverage—limit set in the policy for maximum payment

waiver—"an agreement attached to a policy which exempts from coverage certain disabilities normally covered by the policy"

Hypothetical Example of a Health Insurance Policy. Hospital (coverage) insurance for people under age 65 (age limit) paying 100 dollars a day (benefits) for each day in the hospital up to fifty days (upper limit of coverage). The policy is good for one year (policy term) and excludes treatment for mental illness and tuberculosis (exclusions). Preexisting medical conditions not covered (preexisting conditions), payments due monthly by the fifth day of the month (five-day grace period), and the company must receive notice of hospitalization not less than thirty days after admission to the hospital (time limit).

More Characteristics of Health Insurance Policies

Premium—"the periodic payment required to keep the policy in force"

Indemnity—"a benefit paid by a health insurance policy for an insured loss"

Claim—"a demand by an insured person for benefits provided by a policy"—a request for payment

Non-Cancellable (Guaranteed Renewable) Policy—(Opposite of an "optional renewable policy") "a policy which the insured has the right to continue in force by the timely payment of premiums set forth in the policy to a specified age during which period the insurer has no right to make any change in any provision of the policy while the policy is in force." Usually, the insurer can not change the premium rate for an individual insured person. The insurer may or may not be allowed to make premium rate changes for all similar policyholders.

Group Insurance (as distinct from *Individual* or *Personal Insurance*)— "a policy protecting a group of persons—usually employees for a firm," rather than a policy providing protection to a policyholder and/or family. One difference is that the insurer estimates the expected risk for the group as a whole, rather than for each individual.

Other Types of Benefits

Coinsurance—a policy provision by which both the insured person and the insurance company share the expenses of illness or injury in a specified proportion. (For example, the insurer will pay 80 percent of the hospital bill while the insured pays the remaining 20 percent.)

Deductible—"that portion of covered hospital and medical charges which the insured person must pay before benefits begin." This is in contrast to *first dollar coverage*, where there is no deductible.

Assignment of Benefits (Non-Service Benefits)—Frequently hospitals or other providers of care will have patients assign (transfer) the benefits from the patient to the hospital so that the insurance company pays the hospital directly.

Community vs. Experience Rating of Premiums

In *community rating*, all the people in an area (e.g., a state) would pay the same premium, whether they are young or old, rich or poor, and in spite of the fact that some people have a predictably greater chance of using health care benefits. In this way the high users would not have to pay very high premiums.

In *experience rating*, individuals or groups are charged premiums proportional to their expected level of utilization.

Under competitive conditions, community rating is not possible because other insurers will offer lower premiums to low risk groups, leaving the community rating insurer with the high risk groups.

Multiple Coverage is when an individual has more than one insurance or prepayment policy covering the same event. In this case, he would make money if the event occurred, and therefore this is a question of moral hazard.

Hypothetical Example of Deductible, Coinsurance, Upper Limit and Not Covered Expenses. The hospital bill is $1,000. The insurance policy has a $50 deductible, 10 percent coinsurance and an upper limit of $600. Fifty dollars of the hospital bill is not covered because of exclusions in the policy (uninsured expenses). Diagrammatically this can be represented as follows:[3]

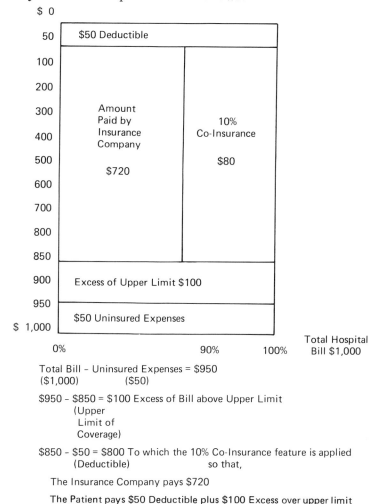

Total Bill – Uninsured Expenses = $950
($1,000)   ($50)

$950 – $850 = $100 Excess of Bill above Upper Limit
        (Upper
        Limit of
        Coverage)

$850 – $50 = $800 To which the 10% Co-Insurance feature is applied
        (Deductible)   so that,

The Insurance Company pays $720

The Patient pays $50 Deductible plus $100 Excess over upper limit plus $50 Uninsured Expenses and $80 Co-Insurance for a total of $280.*

Hypothetical Simplified Example of How Premiums Are Calculated.
Assume the policy is to pay $100 a day (benefit) for each day of hospital care (coverage) for the first 50 days for each admission

[3] Figures are chosen for ease of calculation, not as typical of policies in use.

*Note that if the deductions and co-insurance are removed in a different order, the insurance coverage will vary accordingly. The order of calculation would be defined by the policy.

(upper limit) for the coming year (policy term). It is to cover the 1,000 employees of X Company. The company will pay half the cost and the employees will have the other half deducted from their monthly pay check. By analyzing the previous year's experience of these employees it was found that the average employee used 1.1 hospital days per year, or 1,100 total days for all 1,000 employees. It was also found that the total number of hospital days in excess of the 50 limit was 100 days.

This leaves 1,000 days of hospital care to be covered at $100 a day, or $100,000 yearly in total benefits. To this figure is added 20 percent for administrative expenses, overhead, reserves, profits and so forth, for a total needed revenue of $120,000 per year. Of this the company pays half, $60,000, and each individual employee pays $60 per year or $5 per month—the monthly premium. Modifications in the benefits would make these calculations much more complex. This kind of analysis is carried out by Insurance *actuaries*.

Major Forms of Health Insurance

1. hospital (pays hospital bills)
2. surgical (pays for doctor's operating fees and related care)
3. regular medical (pays for nonsurgical doctor fees in hospital and nonhospital physician care)
4. major medical (pays for all expenses with coinsurance and deductible designed especially to cover major illness)
5. disability (loss of income)

Characteristics of the Insured Event

A major problem for insurers and providers is to make their obligations both predictable and bounded by some upper known limit. The actuaries who design insurance and benefits (and prepayment, as in Blue Cross) consider the following characteristics of the event to be covered. These characteristics play a basic role in defining the extent and type of coverage:

1. The Insured Event should be *unpredictable* or random in the individual case but predictable on average. For example, one cannot predict whether an individual coin toss will come up heads or not, but one does know that there is a 50 percent chance of this happening over many tosses. Thus, the concept of pooling of risks. If the event were predictable, then one would buy insurance on the day of the event and let the policy lapse the day after. (For example, maternity benefits to already pregnant mothers.)

2. The Insured Event should be *definable* so that everyone can agree that it has occurred. For example, a broken leg is definable, but it is not so easy to say when a neurosis calls for psychotherapy.
3. The Insured Event should be *uncontrollable*, like lightning striking a barn. To the extent that events are controllable there is the issue of *moral hazard*; for example, the owner of a failing company who sets fire to the building in order to collect the fire insurance. Because of this problem, insurance usually pays less than the real value of the total loss. In health insurance there is the possible moral hazard of doctors and patients conspiring to use unnecessary health care.
4. The Insured Event should be relatively *large* so that the *administrative costs* of writing the insurance coverage are proportionally small. People have enough money available to cover small events. It is the big costs which may bankrupt them. One reason for a deductible is to avoid the administrative costs of processing small claims.
5. Insured Events should be *independent* events in the statistical sense. Non-independent events are the plague, war, and widespread natural disasters where, if one person is harmed, many others will also be harmed. The large expenditures that would result would bankrupt the insurance company.
6. Expenses connected with the event should be *finite*, known and defined. This allows the insurer to estimate how much he can expect to pay out, and that payments will not be infinitely large. For this reason most insurance policies have upper limits on coverage and some arrangement to insure that they do not have to pay if the doctor charges a very high fee or if the automobile repairman submits an inflated bill.
7. The average predicted value of the Insured Event occurring is small enough so that people will buy the insurance. Insuring 90-year-old men who have already had two heart attacks for $100,000 in event of their death is an example. If they have a 50 percent chance of dying within the year, the premium would be $50,000 excluding administrative costs.

The more the event is characterized by the above, the more appropriate the insurance approach.

In short, insurance is the pooling of risks, but when the insurance company undertakes to cover a risk, it, too, wants to set predictable limits on its commitments.[4]

[4] *Reinsurance* is insuring the insurance company against too great a loss. For example, having the government undertake to pay for an insurer's yearly bene-

One should also distinguish between health insurance and the issue of the equitable distribution of health care (access to health care), i.e., the young paying for the health costs of the old, and the well-to-do paying for the poor.

Provision of Services

This approach, unlike the insurance approach to defining risk above, is to provide a certain fixed level of services for a given population, to be used up to a limit. If there is demand or need in excess of services provided, people may either wait for care (*queue*) or go without. Urban city hospitals for the care of the poor are an example of this approach.

Providers of Private Insurance
(Non-government Agencies)

Blue Cross—"an independent (nongovernment, private) non-profit tax-exempt membership corporation providing protection against the costs of hospital care in a limited geographic area"

Blue Shield—"an independent nonprofit membership corporation providing protection against the costs of surgery and other items of medical care in a limited geographic area"

If there is a single starting point for Blue Cross, it was the prepayment plan for Dallas teachers established at Baylor University by Justin F. Kimball in 1929. The American Hospital Association endorsed this prepayment idea in 1933. The next year the Blue Cross symbol was first used to designate non-profit hospital plans. By 1938, the basic principles for Blue Cross plans were established.

1. They are non-profit organizations.
2. Board of Directors are to represent hospitals, physicians, and the public.
3. They are to be supervised by state insurance departments.
4. Hold low cash reserves.
5. Emphasis on hospital benefits in the form of service, rather than cash indemnities.
6. Plans are not to be in competition with each other, and therefore do not have overlapping geographical boundries.

---

fits if they exceed an agreed-upon limit beyond which the insurer, if he had to pay it by himself, would go bankrupt.

7. Employees are on salary and salesmen are not paid on commission.

By 1937, the State medical societies of California, Michigan, and Pennsylvania were sponsoring physician service plans. In 1946, the AMA financed the Associated Medical Care Plans, which became the National Association of Blue Shield Plans.

By 1960, the Blue Cross Association became the sole national federation of Blue Cross plans.[5]

Blue Cross and Blue Shield (the Blues, or BC-BS, or BX) are legally independent of each other, but often work in close cooperation with each other in offering matched benefit packages to insured groups.

There are approximately seventy Blue Cross organizations covering part of a state (Associated Hospital Service of New York), an entire state (Massachusetts Blue Cross), or several states (Vermont and New Hampshire).

They are linked as members of the Blue Cross Association which provides shared services and arranges for coverage with other Blue Cross plans for travelers who leave their own plan's area.

Blue Cross is set up in most states under special enabling legislation, generally providing that it should be regulated by the state insurance department. In some states Blue Cross must submit to public hearings before it can raise its rates.

Up to 1972 the American Hospital Association owned the Blue Cross symbol and set requirements for corporations using this symbol, including (a) it cover a large enough area, (b) provide service benefits, (c) should have a contract with the majority of hospitals in its area, and (d) have at least one-third of the board representing the public and one-third representing the contracting hospitals.

Blue Cross calls these features which distinguish it from other private insurance companies "prepayment" rather than "insurance." *Service benefits* (as opposed to direct (cash) payments to insured persons to pay for care, which are called *indemnity benefits*) consist of "a contract benefit which is paid directly to the provider of hospital or medical care for services rendered."

This requires a contractual agreement between the insurer and provider of care (hospitals and Blue Cross, doctors and Blue Shield) and distinguishes the Blue Cross, Blue Shield plans from the com-

[5] Odin Anderson. *Blue Cross Since 1929.* Ballinger Publishing Company, Cambridge, Massachusetts, 1975.

mercial insurers who make payments to the (beneficiary) patient, not the provider.

The Blue Cross contract usually specifies what the hospital is allowed to charge the patients covered by Blue Cross. The hospitals are not limited in this way with patients covered by commercial insurance policies.

Blue Cross Enabling Legislation at the State Level.   Although the contents of this legislation varies from state to state, it usually includes the following:

a. Blue Cross and Blue Shield are allowed to operate in the state.
b. The state insurance commissioner is given certain powers to regulate the plan.
c. Premium rate increases must be approved by the insurance commissioner after a public hearing.
d. Blue Cross and Blue Shield are the only organizations which are allowed to contract with providers for service benefits at agreed-upon charges.

Private Insurance Companies.[6]   Several hundred companies write health insurance, using thousands of different policies. Some major companies include Prudential, Equitable, Aetna, Metropolitan, and Connecticut General.

Independent (Private Insurance) Plans.   These plans include:

Kaiser-Permanente Plan
Health Insurance Plan of Greater New York (HIP)
Various union-sponsored plans

These are generally in the form of prepaid group practice.

Workmen's Compensation started in the first decade of this century. By 1948 all states had workmen's compensation, in addition to the Federal Employees Compensation Act (FECA, passed in 1908, replaced in 1916, and amended in 1949 by PL 81-357), and the Longshoremen and Harbor Workers Act. These laws are based on the idea that the employer is financially liable for injuries to employees,

---

[6] These are sometimes called *commercial insurance companies.* The word "commercial" is not used by the companies in this category and has ideological implications related to the competition between these companies and Blue Cross and Blue Shield.

although the employee does not have to prove that the employer was negligent.

There are three categories of benefits: (a) cash, (b) medical, and (c) rehabilitation to indemnify the worker injured on the job or his dependents for loss of wages, medical and hospital expenses, and loss of occupational capacity and skills.

These benefits are financed by employers, either through insuring with a private insurance company or, in some states, through a state fund or by self-insurance. Benefits vary substantially from state to state and by type of employment.

References

Health Insurance Institute, *Source Book of Health Insurance Data*, New York, Yearly (Quotations from this source).

American Hospital Association, *Approval Program for Blue Cross Plans* (Chicago: The Association, 1964).

Health/PAC Bulletin, "Health Research Guide," New York, No. 28, February 1971.

O.D. Dickerson, *Health Insurance* (Homewood, Illinois: Richard D. Irwin, Inc., 1959).

H.M. Somers and A.R. Somers, *Workman's Compensation* (New York: John Wiley & Sons, 1954).

3. HEALTH PLANS, HMOs

Health plans include *Health Maintenance Organization* (HMOs) and *Prepaid Group Practice* (PGP). HMO is the more general term. In fact, it is often so general as to be difficult to define. HMOs include Prepaid Group Practice and *Foundations for Medical Care* (FMC), which are described under ambulatory care.

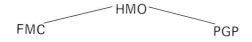

Characteristics of HMOs include the following:

1. It provides directly, or through arrangement with other health services, to enrollees on a per capita prepayment basis. Thus it

has a defined population being served. Each enrollee pays a fixed amount, regardless of the volume of services he uses.

2. The HMO provides physician services through physicians who are partners or employees, or through a contractual arrangement with a group of physicians.
3. The services provided are comprehensive, that is, covering a range of services, usually including inpatient and outpatient care.
4. There are internal, self-regulating mechanisms to assure quality of care and cost control. An organization is responsible for the health care of the population served.

Thus, HMOs combine the provision of service, the barring or risk (insurance or prepayment), and performance monitoring. For many people, one of the ideas behind HMOs is that HMO doctors will be responsible for the hospital bill incurred when they admit a patient to the hospital and, therefore, the HMO doctors will be careful not to admit patients unnecessarily.

Prepaid Group Practice or *Comprehensive Prepaid Group Practice* refers to an HMO where services are provided by doctors in organized group practice. PGPs may or may not own their own hospitals. (For example, Kaiser does and GHI and HIP do not.)

Some of the well-known PGPs include

GHI (Group Health Association of Washington, D.C.)
Group Health Cooperative of Puget Sound (Washington)
Harvard Community Health Plan (Boston)
HIP (Health Insurance Plan of Greater New York)
HMO International (Los Angeles)
Kaiser-Permanente
Ross-Loos Medical Group (Los Angeles)

Although it has many distinctive features when compared with other plans, Kaiser-Permanente, the largest and most frequently cited example, will be described here.

Kaiser-Permanente. This is the largest, nongovernmental *prepaid group practice* health plan in the country. Permanente Medical Groups and the Kaiser Foundation Hospitals are two separate corporate entities working closely together to provide

a. a nongovernment (private),
b. prepaid (fixed monthly payments by members regardless of use of services),
c. group practice (three or more doctors practicing together and sharing income),

d. nonprofit,
e. comprehensive health plan (provides a wide range of doctor, hospital and ancillary services) serving an identifiable population (consumer groups and individuals).

The plan was started to take care of the employees of Kaiser Industries prior to World War II and was opened to the public just after the war. By 1970 it served 2.1 million members in California, Oregon, Washington, Hawaii, Colorado, and Ohio. Most members are enrolled according to their place of employment (group employment).

Physicians are members or partners of the Permanente Medical Groups. The Kaiser Foundation Hospitals own and operate their facilities. Emphasis is placed on outpatient rather than inpatient services. Doctors' offices are usually in or near the hospital and physicians are salaried. In some parts of Kaiser-Permanente, part of any surplus revenue generated by the plan is returned to physicians so there is a financial incentive here for them to keep total costs down. The plan has a lower admission rate per 1,000 population to hospitals in comparison to adjacent Blue Cross-Blue Shield subscribers.

References

Greer Williams, *Kaiser-Permanente Health Plan: Why It Works* (The Henry Kaiser Foundation, 300 Lakeside Drive, Oakland, California 94604, 1971).

Report of the National Advisory Commission on Health Manpower (Washington, D.C.: U.S. Government Printing Office, November 1967), Vol. II, Appendix IV.

"Kaiser-Permanente—Controversial Plan in News," *American Medical News*, September 13, 1971.

Anne R. Somers (editor), *The Kaiser-Permanente Medical Care Program: A Symposium* (New York: The Commonwealth Fund, 1971).

4. FINANCING

The Flow of Funds for the Provision of Health Care

Customarily, payments for health insurance and Medicare Part A are made in relationship to place of employment. The employee and employer pay taxes and Social Security payments (employer contribution and employee's *payroll deduction*). Insurance, Blue Cross, or other coverage for the employee and his family (dependents) is also customarily obtained at the place of employment (*employee benefit plans*). The employee pays through payroll deductions and the employer usually contributes to the premium as a *fringe benefit*. (Fringe benefits are non-salary compensations, such as health and life insurance, retirement benefits, etc.) Blue Cross provides payments directly to the provider (vendor) in the form of service benefits. These providers are under contract. Insurance companies have no contractual arrangement with providers (usually this is forbidden by state insurance laws). Insurance companies pay benefits directly to the subscriber who, in turn, pays the provider. The subscriber may *assign* his benefits to the provider and then the insurance company will send its benefit directly to the provider. In addition, there are *out-of-pocket* (or direct) expenses paid directly by the user to the provider.

Finally, there are some unemployed, uninsured, and/or indigent persons who make no payments for the care they receive.

Government expenditures are (at the federal, state, and local levels) both for services provided (government hospitals, for example) and for payment to non-governmental providers (*vendor payments*). In this context, government, Blue Cross-Blue Shield, and insurance companies are referred to as *third party payers* (the other "parties" being patient and provider).

The agreement between providers (usually hospitals) and third party payers (usually Blue Cross, and government programs) as to what will be paid for and how much is called the *reimbursement formula*. These can be exceedingly complicated. For example, "cost or charges, whichever is less" means that the third party payer will pay either the provider's actual costs, or what it ordinarily charges patients, whichever figure is lower.

Prospective reimbursement means that the payer and the provider agree in advance on a budget for the provider and, therefore, on the provider's expected costs. If the provider's services cost more, then the provider must absorb the loss. If the provider's services cost less, the provider keeps the extra. This, and other formulae which try to encourage efficient provider performance, is called *incentive reimbursement*.

Preadmission (Prospective) Screening of Admissions means that the doctor and/or hospital must receive prior approval from the payer to admit an elective patient, in order to be reimbursed.

Retrospective Denial of Payment means that the payer reviews the appropriateness of the use of services, after they have been used.

If the payer finds the services provided were medically unnecessary, it will not reimburse the provider for them.

National Health Expenditure Data

As the charts and tables on pages 104–115 indicate:

1. National health expenditures have been rising and include a growing share of the *gross national product* (the value of all goods and services produced in the country during the year).
2. The proportion of health care expenditures paid by the government has been increasing.
3. Federal health expenditures are greater than state and local expenditures.
4. Type of payment varies by the type of service provided.

Need and Demand for Care

Need for care—This usually refers to an expert estimate of the health services a person or population requires.

Unmet need—The difference between *realized demand* and *need*

Realized demand—The amount of health care actually used

Demand—(a) Medical care definition: The amount of care that people would use if there were no barriers to use (like cost or access); (b) Economic definition: The amount of care purchased at a given price.

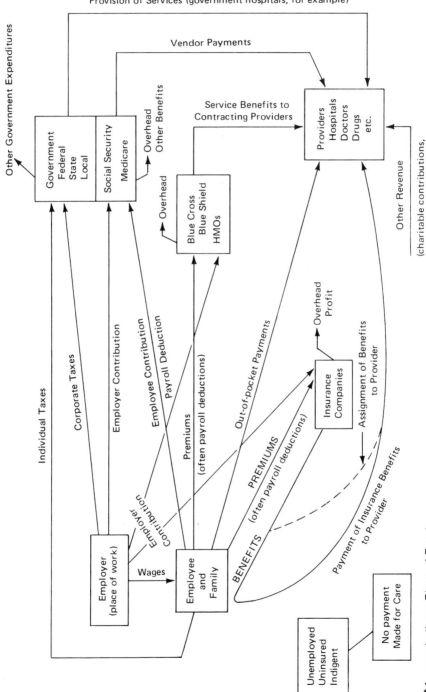

Grants for Research or Special Projects
Payment for Services (Medicaid, for example)
Provision of Services (government hospitals, for example)

Vendor Payments

Service Benefits to
Contracting Providers

Other Government Expenditures

Government
Federal
State
Local

Social Security
Medicare

Overhead
Other Benefits

Providers
Hospitals
Doctors
Drugs
etc.

Other Revenue
(charitable contributions,
for example)

Overhead

Blue Cross
Blue Shield
HMOs

Individual Taxes

Corporate Taxes

Employer Contribution

Employee Contribution
Payroll Deduction

Premiums
(often payroll deductions)

Out-of-pocket Payments

Overhead
Profit

Insurance
Companies

Assignment of Benefits
to Provider

PREMIUMS
(often payroll deductions)

Payment of Insurance Benefits
to Provider

BENEFITS

Employer
Contribution

Employer
(place of work)

Wages

Employee
and
Family

Unemployed
Uninsured
Indigent

No payment
Made for Care

*Arrows indicate Flow of Funds.

Figure 3-1. Payment for Health Services: Schematic Diagram of Flow of Funds* (Simplified).

104

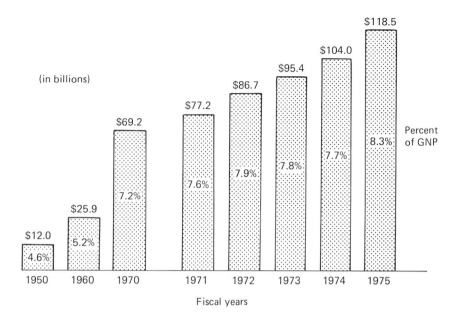

Figure 3-2. National Health Expenditures and Percentage of Gross National Product, Selected Fiscal Years, 1950-75.

Source: Marjorie Smith Mueller and Robert M. Gibson, "National Health Expenditures, Fiscal Year 1975," *Social Security Bulletin* 39, 2 (February 1976).

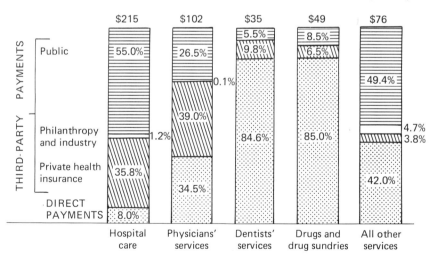

Figure 3-3. Distribution of Personal Health Care Expenditures, by Source of Funds and Type of Expenditures, Fiscal Year 1975.

Source: Marjorie Smith Mueller and Robert M. Gibson, "National Health Expenditures, Fiscal Year 1975," *Social Security Bulletin* 39, 2 (February 1976).

Table 3-1.   Aggregate and Per Capita National Health Expenditures, by Source of Funds, and Percentage of Gross National Product, Selected Fiscal Years, 1929 through 1975

Fiscal year	Gross national product (in billions)	Health expenditures								
		Total			Private			Public		
		Amount (in millions)	Per capita	Percent of GNP	Amount (in millions)	Per capita	Percent of total	Amount (in millions)	Per capita	Percent of total
1929	$101.0	$3,589	$29.16	3.6	$3,112	$25.28	86.7	$477	$3.88	13.3
1935	68.7	2,846	22.04	4.1	2,303	17.84	80.9	543	4.21	19.1
1940	95.1	3,863	28.83	4.1	3,081	22.99	79.8	782	5.84	20.2
1950	263.4	12,028	78.35	4.6	8,962	58.38	74.5	3,065	19.97	25.5
1955	379.7	17,330	103.76	4.6	12,909	77.29	74.5	4,421	26.46	25.5
1960	495.6	25,856	141.63	5.2	19,461	106.60	75.3	6,395	35.03	24.7
1965	655.6	38,892	197.75	5.9	29,357	149.27	75.5	9,535	48.48	24.5
1966	718.5	42,109	211.56	5.9	31,279	157.15	74.3	10,830	54.41	25.7
1967	771.4	47,879	237.93	6.2	32,057	159.30	67.0	15,823	78.63	33.0
1968	827.0	53,765	264.37	6.5	33,727	165.84	62.7	20,040	98.54	37.3
1969	899.0	60,617	295.20	6.7	37,682	183.51	62.2	22,937	111.70	37.8
1970	954.8	69,202	333.57	7.2	43,964	211.92	63.5	25,238	121.65	36.5
1971	1,013.6	77,162	368.25	7.6	48,558	231.74	62.9	28,604	136.51	37.1
1972	1,100.6	86,687	409.71	7.9	53,398	252.37	61.6	33,289	157.33	38.4
1973	1,225.2	95,384	447.31	7.8	58,995	276.66	61.8	36,389	170.65	38.2
1974	1,348.9	104,030	484.53	7.7	62,152	294.03	60.7	40,879	190.33	39.3
1975[1]	1,424.3	118,500	547.03	8.3	68,552	316.46	57.8	49,948	230.57	42.2

1. Preliminary estimates.

Source: Marjorie Smith Mueller and Robert M. Gibson, "National Health Expenditures, Fiscal Year 1975," *Social Security Bulletin* 39, 2 (February 1976).

Table 3-2. National Health Expenditures, by Type of Expenditure and Source of Funds, Fiscal Years, 1973–75 [In millions]

Type of expenditure	Total	Source of funds					
		Private			*Public*		
		Total	*Consumers*	*Other*	*Total*	*Federal*	*State and local*
				1975[1]			
Total	$118,500	$68,552	$63,784	$4,768	$49,948	$33,828	$16,119
Health services and supplies	111,250	65,665	63,784	1,881	45,585	30,776	14,808
Hospital care	46,600	20,957	20,413	544	25,643	18,264	7,380
Physicians' services	22,100	16,245	16,230	15	5,855	4,262	1,593
Dentists' services	7,500	7,085	7,085	—	415	255	160
Other professional services	2,100	1,591	1,551	40	509	342	167
Drugs and drug sundries	10,600	9,695	9,695	—	905	478	427
Eyeglasses and appliances	2,300	2,198	2,198	—	102	57	45
Nursing-home care	9,000	3,799	3,767	32	5,201	2,982	2,220
Expenses for prepayment and administration	4,953	3,389	2,845	544	1,204	997	207
Government public health activities	3,457	—	—	—	3,457	1,201	2,256
Other health services	3,000	706	—	706	2,294	1,939	355
Research and medical-facilities construction	7,250	2,887	—	2,887	4,363	3,052	1,311
Research[2]	2,750	235	—	235	2,515	2,418	97
Construction	4,500	2,652	—	2,652	1,848	634	1,214
Publicly owned facilities	1,266	—	—	—	1,266	68	1,198
Privately owned facilities	3,234	2,652	—	2,652	582	566	16
				1974[3]			
Total	$104,030	$63,152	$58,224	$4,928	$40,879	$27,484	$13,395
Health services and supplies	97,214	59,972	58,224	1,748	37,243	24,913	12,330
Hospital care	39,963	18,639	18,126	513	21,324	14,626	6,698

(continued)

Table 3-2.   National Health Expenditures, by Type of Expenditure and Source of Funds, Fiscal Years, 1973-75 [In millions]

Type of expenditure	Total	Source of funds					
		Private			Public		
		Total	Consumers	Other	Total	Federal	State and local
Physicians' services	19,571	14,834	14,820	14	4,737	3,420	1,318
Dentists' services	6,783	6,450	6,450	—	333	215	118
Other professional services	1,927	1,576	1,538	38	351	225	126
Drugs and drug sundries[2]	9,612	8,862	8,862	—	750	410	340
Eyeglasses and appliances	2,160	2,070	2,070	—	90	50	40
Nursing-home care	7,450	3,574	3,544	30	3,876	2,314	1,562
Expenses for prepayment and administration	4,501	3,342	2,814	528	1,159	995	164
Government public health activities	2,625	—	—	—	2,625	959	1,666
Other health services	2,622	625	—	625	1,997	1,699	298
Research and medical-facilities construction	6,816	3,180	—	3,180	3,636	2,571	1,065
Research[2]	2,389	219	—	219	2,170	2,078	92
Construction	4,427	2,961	—	2,961	1,466	493	973
Publicly owned facilities	1,167	—	—	—	1,167	209	958
Privately owned facilities	3,260	2,961	—	2,961	299	284	15
				1973[3]			
Total	$ 95,384	$58,995	$54,213	$4,782	$36,389	$24,280	$21,109
Health services and supplies	88,941	55,846	54,213	1,633	33,095	21,793	11,302
Hospital care	36,155	17,113	16,642	471	19,042	12,793	6,249
Physicians' services	17,995	13,861	13,849	12	4,134	3,008	1,126
Dentists' services	6,101	5,780	5,780	—	321	218	104
Other professional services	1,781	1,440	1,406	34	341	224	117
Drugs and drug sundries[2]	8,987	8,272	8,272	—	715	387	328
Eyeglasses and appliances	1,986	1,905	1,905	—	81	45	35
Nursing-home care	6,650	3,477	3,449	28	3,173	1,849	1,323

Expenses for prepayment and administration	4,299	3,418	2,910	508	881	704	177
Government public health activities	2,152	—	—	—	2,152	911	1,241
Other health services	2,835	580	—	580	2,255	1,654	601
Research and medical-facilities construction	6,443	3,149	—	3,149	3,294	2,487	807
Research[2]	2,298	208	—	208	2,090	2,002	88
Construction	4,145	2,941	—	2,941	1,204	485	719
Publicly owned facilities	967	—	—	—	967	262	705
Privately owned facilities	3,178	2,941	—	2,941	237	223	14

1. Preliminary estimates.

2. Research expenditures of drug companies in "drugs and drug sundries" excluded from "research expenditures."

3. Revised estimates.

Source: Marjorie Smith Mueller and Robert M. Gibson, "National Health Expenditures, Fiscal Year 1975," *Social Security Bulletin* 39, 2 (February 1976).

Table 3-3. Expenditures for Health Services and Supplies under Public Programs, by Program, Type of Expenditures, and Source of Funds, Fiscal Year 1973-75 [In millions]

Program and source of funds	Total	Hospital care	Physicians' services	Dentists' services	Other professional services	Drugs and drug sundries	Eye glasses and appliances	Nursing-home care	Government public health activities	Other health services	Administration
Total	$45,584.7	$25,643.3	$5,855.4	$414.8	$508.7	$904.6	$102.2	$5,201.3	$3,457.0	$2,293.6	$1,203.8
Health insurance for aged and disabled[2,3]	14,781.4	10,710.6	2,967.1	—	186.1	—	—	257.0	—	—	660.6
Temporary disability insurance (medical benefits)[2]	73.3	53.6	17.0	—	1.2	0.8	0.7	—	—	—	—
Workmen's compensation (medical benefits)[4]	1,830.0	922.6	777.7	—	56.4	36.6	36.7	—	—	—	—
Public assistance (vendor medical payments)[3]	12,968.0	4,270.5	1,685.7	337.1	224.8	836.6	—	4,782.4	—	349.7	481.2
General hospital and medical care	5,491.7	5,369.7	13.9	3.2	—	1.6	—	—	—	103.3	—
Defense Department hospital and medical care (including military dependents)[5]	3,011.0	1,903.8	216.8	10.8	—	9.7	—	—	—	848.3	21.6
Maternal and child health services	540.0	81.9	49.8	12.3	40.2	11.8	16.1	—	—	323.3	4.6
School health[6]	—	—	—	—	—	—	—	—	—	—	—
Other public Health activities	—	—	—	—	—	—	—	—	3,457.0	—	—
Veterans' hospital and medical care	3,242.3	2,253.6	32.4	51.4	—	7.5	30.7	161.9	—	669.0	35.8
Medical vocational rehabilitation[7]	190.0	77.0	95.0	—	—	—	18.0	—	—	—	—
Office of Economic Opportunity[7]	—	—	—	—	—	—	—	—	—	—	—
Federal	30,776.3	18,263.5	4,262.3	254.8	342.0	477.6	57.1	2,981.8	1,201.0	1,939.0	997.2
Health insurance for aged and disabled[2,3]	14,781.4	10,710.6	2,967.1	—	186.1	—	—	257.0	—	—	660.6
Workmen's compensation (medical benefits)	50.6	32.9	12.6	—	3.0	1.0	1.1	—	—	—	—
Public assistance (vendor medical payments)[5]	6,966.4	2,288.6	903.4	180.7	120.5	448.3	—	2,562.9	—	187.4	274.6
General hospital and medical care	1,089.5	967.6	13.9	3.2	—	1.6	—	—	—	103.3	—
Defense Department hospital and medical care (including military dependents)[5]	3,011.0	1,903.8	216.8	10.8	—	9.7	—	—	—	848.3	21.6
Maternal and child health services	277.0	42.8	37.6	8.7	32.4	9.5	10.4	—	—	131.0	4.6
Other public health activities	1,201.0	—	—	—	—	—	—	—	1,201.0	—	—
Veterans' hospital and medical care[5]	3,242.3	2,253.6	32.4	51.4	—	7.5	30.7	161.9	—	669.0	35.8
Medical vocational rehabilitation[7]	157.0	63.6	78.5	—	—	—	14.9	—	—	—	—
Office of Economic Opportunity[7]	—	—	—	—	—	—	—	—	—	—	—

State and local	14,808.4	7,379.8	1,593.1	160.1	166.7	427.0	45.1	2,219.5	2,256.0	354.5	206.6
Temporary disability insurance (medical benefits)[2,4]	73.3	53.6	17.0	—	1.2	0.8	0.7	—	—	—	—
Workmen's compensation (medical benefits)[4]	1,779.4	889.7	765.1	—	53.4	35.6	35.6	—	—	—	—
Public assistance (vendor medical payments)[5]	6,001.7	1,981.9	782.3	156.5	104.3	388.3	—	2,219.5	—	162.2	206.6
General hospital and medical care	4,402.1	4,402.1	—	—	—	—	—	—	—	—	—
Maternal and child health services	263.0	39.1	12.2	3.6	7.8	2.3	5.7	—	—	192.3	—
School health[6]	—	—	—	—	—	—	—	—	—	—	—
Other public health activities	2,256.0	—	—	—	—	—	—	—	2,256.0	—	—
Medical vocational rehabilitation	33.0	13.4	16.5	—	—	3.1	3.1	—	—	—	—
Total	$37,242.6	$21,324.1	$4,737.4	$332.8	$351.0	$750.3	$89.9	$3,876.3	$2,625.3	$1,997.0	$1,158.5
						1974[3]					
Health insurance for aged and disabled[2,3]	11,347.5	8,049.1	2,321.9	—	106.3	—	—	203.0	—	—	667.2
Temporary disability insurance (medical benefits)[4]	70.7	52.0	16.1	—	1.1	0.8	0.7	—	—	—	—
Workmen's compensation (medical benefits)[4]	1,560.0	785.5	664.3	—	47.9	31.2	31.1	—	—	—	—
Public assistance (vendor medical payments)[3]	10,371.9	3,617.6	1,401.3	258.4	159.0	695.7	—	3,548.0	—	258.4	433.5
General hospital and medical care	5,061.0	4,965.5	11.5	3.8	—	1.6	—	—	—	78.6	—
Defense Department hospital and medical care (including military dependents)[5]	2,741.0	1,738.3	157.6	14.5	—	4.5	—	—	—	803.8	22.3
Maternal and child health services[6]	493.4	74.8	45.5	11.2	36.7	10.8	14.7	—	—	295.2	4.5
School health[6]	—	—	—	—	—	—	—	—	—	—	—
Other public health activities	2,625.3	—	—	—	—	—	—	—	2,625.3	—	—
Veterans' hospital and medical care	2,786.6	1,967.2	25.8	44.9	—	5.7	25.7	125.3	—	561.0	31.0
Medical vocational rehabilitation	185.2	74.1	93.4	—	—	—	17.7	—	—	—	—
Office of Economic Opportunity[7]	—	—	—	—	—	—	—	—	—	—	—
Federal	24,913.2	14,626.4	3,419.7	215.3	224.9	409.9	49.9	2,314.5	959.0	1,698.8	994.8
Health insurance for aged and disabled[2,3]	11,347.5	8,049.1	2,321.9	—	106.3	—	—	203.0	—	—	667.2
Workmen's compensation (medical benefits)	36.1	23.5	9.0	—	2.2	0.7	—	—	—	—	—
Public assistance (vendor medical payments)[5]	5,833.2	2,025.1	784.5	144.7	89.0	389.4	—	1,986.2	—	144.6	269.8
General hospital and medical care	821.0	725.5	11.5	3.8	—	1.6	—	—	—	78.6	—
Defense Department hospital and medical care (including military dependents)[5]	2,741.0	1,738.3	157.6	14.5	—	4.5	—	—	—	803.8	22.3

Table 3-3 continued

Program and source of funds	Total	Hospital care	Physicians' services	Dentists' services	Other professional services	Drugs and drug sundries	Eye glasses and appliances	Nursing-home care	Government public health activities	Other health services	Administration
Maternal and child health services	234.7	36.1	31.8	7.4	27.4	80	8.7	—	—	110.8	4.5
Other public health activities	959.0	—	—	—	—	—	—	—	959.0	—	—
Veterans' hospital and medical care[5]	2,786.6	1,967.2	25.8	44.9	—	5.7	25.7	125.3	—	561.0	31.0
Medical vocational rehabilitation[7]	154.0	61.6	77.6	—	—	—	14.8	—	—	—	—
Office of Economic Opportunity[7]	—	—	—	—	—	—	—	—	—	—	—
State and local	12,329.5	6,697.7	1,317.8	117.5	126.1	340.3	40.0	1,561.8	1,666.3	298.2	163.8
Temporary disability insurance (medical benefits)[4]	70.7	52.0	16.1	—	1.1	0.8	0.7	—	—	—	—
Workmen's compensation (medical benefits)[4]	1,523.9	762.0	655.3	—	45.7	30.5	30.4	—	—	—	—
Public assistance (vendor medical payments)[3]	4,358.7	1,592.5	616.9	113.7	70.0	306.2	—	1,561.8	—	113.8	163.8
General hospital and medical care	4,240.0	4,240.0	—	—	—	—	—	—	—	—	—
Maternal and child health services[4]	258.7	38.7	13.7	3.8	9.3	2.8	6.0	—	—	184.4	—
School health[6]	—	—	—	—	—	—	—	—	—	—	—
Other public health activities	1,666.3	—	—	—	—	—	—	—	1,666.3	—	—
Medical vocational rehabilitation	31.2	12.5	15.8	—	—	—	2.9	—	—	—	—
1973[8]											
Total	$33,094.5	$19,042.0	$4,134.3	$321.4	$340.8	$714.6	$80.8	$3,172.6	$2,151.7	$2,255.1	$881.1
Health insurance for aged[2,3]	9,478.3	6,768.2	2,015.9	—	83.0	—	—	173.0	—	—	438.7
Temporary disability insurance (medical benefits)[4]	69.8	52.0	15.3	—	1.1	0.7	0.7	—	—	—	—
Workmen's compensation (medical benefits)[4]	1,335.0	672.4	568.3	—	41.0	26.6	26.7	—	—	—	—
Public assistance (vendor medical payments)[5]	9,208.7	3,474.0	1,137.4	220.4	149.9	652.5	—	2,892.1	—	291.0	391.3
General hospital and medical care	4,712.5	4,624.1	8.5	2.2	—	1.3	—	—	—	76.4	—
Defense Department hospital and medical care (including military dependents)[5]	2,468.0	1,548.0	159.7	25.6	33.8	6.4	13.5	—	—	708.0	20.3
Maternal and child health services[6]	455.3	68.9	41.9	10.4	—	10.0	—	—	—	272.1	4.7
School health	300.0	—	—	—	—	—	—	—	—	300.0	—
Other public health activities	2,151.7	—	—	—	—	—	—	—	2,151.7	—	—
Veterans' hospital and medical care	2,587.3	1,767.3	21.6	55.2	—	4.9	23.0	107.5	—	581.7	26.1
Medical vocational rehabilitation	175.0	67.1	91.0	—	—	—	16.9	—	—	—	—
Office of Economic Opportunity[7]	152.4	—	74.7	7.6	32.0	12.2	—	—	—	25.9	—

Federal	21,792.9	12,792.8	3,008.0	217.7	223.9	386.9	45.4	1,849.2	911.0	1,653.7	704.3
Health insurance for aged[2,3]	9,478.8	6,768.2	2,015.9	—	83.0	—	—	173.0	—	—	438.7
Workmen's compensation (medical benefits)[5]	32.3	21.0	8.1	—	1.9	0.6	0.7	—	—	—	—
Public assistance (vendor medical payments)[5]	4,997.4	1,884.3	616.9	119.6	81.3	353.9	—	1,568.7	—	158.2	214.5
General hospital and medical care	804.7	716.3	8.5	2.2	—	1.3	—	—	—	76.4	—
Defense Department hospital and medical care (including military dependents)[5]	2,468.0	1,548.0	159.7	25.6	—	6.4	—	—	—	708.0	20.3
Maternal and child health services	221.0	34.0	29.8	7.5	25.7	7.6	8.2	—	—	103.5	4.7
Other public health activities	911.0	—	—	—	—	—	—	—	911.0	—	—
Veterans' hospital and medical care[5]	2,587.3	1,767.3	21.6	55.2	—	4.9	23.0	107.5	—	581.7	26.1
Medical vocational rehabilitation	140.0	53.7	72.8	—	—	—	13.5	—	—	—	—
Office of Economic Opportunity[7]	152.4	—	74.7	7.6	32.0	12.2	—	—	—	25.9	—
State and local	11,301.6	6,249.2	1,126.3	103.8	116.9	327.7	35.4	1,323.4	1,240.7	601.4	176.8
Temporary disability insurance (medical benefits)[3]	69.8	52.0	15.3	—	1.1	0.7	0.7	—	—	—	—
Workmen's compensation (medical benefits)[4]	1,302.7	651.4	560.2	—	39.1	26.0	26.0	—	—	—	—
Public assistance (vendor medical payments)[3]	4,211.3	1,589.7	520.5	100.9	68.6	298.6	—	1,323.4	—	132.8	176.8
General hospital and medical care	3,907.8	3,907.8	—	—	—	—	—	—	—	—	—
Maternal and child health services	234.3	34.9	12.1	2.9	8.1	2.4	5.3	—	—	168.6	—
School health[6]	300.0	—	—	—	—	—	—	—	—	300.0	—
Other public health activities	1,240.7	—	—	—	—	—	—	—	—	—	—
Medical vocational rehabilitation	35.0	13.4	18.2	—	—	—	3.4	—	—	—	—

1. Preliminary estimates.

2. Includes premium payments for supplementary medical insurance by or in behalf of enrollees.

3. Includes duplication in the Medicare and Medicaid amounts where premium payments for Medicare are financed by Medicaid for cash assistance recipients and, in some States, for the medically indigent.

4. Includes medical benefits paid under public law by private insurance carriers and self-insurers.

5. Payments for services outside the hospital (excluding "other health services") represent only those made under contract medical care programs.

6. Beginning in 1974, data not separable from total education expenditures.

7. Beginning in 1974, included with "other public health activities."

8. Revised estimates.

Source: Marjorie Smith Mueller and Robert M. Gibson, "National Health Expenditures, Fiscal Year 1975," Social Security Bulletin 39, 2 (February 1976).

Table 3-4. Aggregate and Per Capita National Health Expenditures, by Type of Expenditure, Selected Fiscal Years, 1929 through 1975

Type of expenditure	Aggregate amount (in millions)							
	1929	1935	1940	1950	1960	1965	1966	1967
Total	$3,589	$2,846	$3,863	$12,027	$25,856	$38,892	$42,109	$47,879
Health services and supplies	3,382	2,788	3,729	11,181	24,162	35,664	38,661	44,343
Hospital care	651	731	969	3,698	8,499	13,152	14,245	16,921
Physicians' services	994	744	946	2,689	5,580	8,405	8,865	9,738
Dentists' services	476	298	402	940	1,944	2,728	2,866	3,158
Other professional services	248	150	173	384	848	989	1,140	1,139
Drugs and drug sundries	601	471	621	1,642	3,591	4,647	5,032	5,480
Eyeglasses and appliances	131	128	180	475	750	1,151	1,309	1,514
Nursing-home care	—	—	28	178	480	1,271	1,407	1,751
Expenses for prepayment and administration	101	91	161	290	807	1,234	1,446	1,818
Government public health activities	89	112	155	351	401	671	731	884
Other health services	90	63	92	534	1,262	1,416	1,620	1,940
Research and medical-facilities construction	207	58	134	847	1,694	3,228	3,448	3,536
Research	—	—	3	110	592	1,391	1,545	1,606
Construction	207	58	131	737	1,102	1,837	1,903	1,930

Type of expenditure	1968	1969	1970	1971	1972[1]	1973[1]	1974[1]	1975[2]
Total	$53,766	$60,617	$69,202	$77,162	$86,687	$95,384	$104,030	$118,500
Health services and supplies	49,802	56,327	64,065	71,762	80,548	88,941	97,214	111,250
Hospital care	19,384	22,356	25,879	29,133	32,720	36,155	39,963	46,600
Physicians' services	10,734	11,842	13,443	15,098	16,527	17,995	19,571	22,100
Dentists' services	3,518	3,920	4,473	4,908	5,364	6,101	6,783	7,500
Other professional services	1,217	1,298	1,385	1,509	1,634	1,781	1,927	2,100
Drugs and drug sundries	5,865	6,482	7,114	7,626	8,239	8,987	9,612	10,600
Eyeglasses and appliances	1,665	1,743	1,776	1,810	1,878	1,986	2,160	2,300
Nursing-home care	2,360	3,057	3,818	4,890	5,860	6,650	7,450	9,000
Expenses for prepayment and administration	1,939	2,066	2,115	2,405	3,645	4,299	4,501	4,593
Government public health activities	1,001	1,195	1,437	1,698	2,075	2,152	2,625	3,457
Other health services	2,119	2,368	2,625	2,685	2,606	2,835	2,622	3,000
Research and medical-facilities construction	3,964	4,290	5,137	5,400	6,139	6,443	6,816	7,250
Research	1,800	1,790	1,846	1,850	2,058	2,298	2,389	2,750
Construction	2,164	2,500	3,291	3,550	4,081	4,145	4,427	4,500

Per capita amount[3]

Type of expenditure	1929	1935	1940	1950	1960	1965	1966	1967
Total	$29.16	$22.04	$28.83	$78.35	$141.63	$197.75	$211.56	$237.93
Health services and supplies	27.48	21.59	27.83	72.83	132.35	181.34	194.24	220.36
Hospital care	5.29	5.66	7.23	24.09	46.56	66.87	71.57	84.09
Physicians' services	8.08	5.76	7.06	17.52	30.57	42.74	44.54	48.39
Dentists' services	3.87	2.31	3.00	6.12	10.65	13.87	14.40	15.69
Other professional services	2.01	1.16	1.29	2.50	4.65	5.03	5.73	5.66
Drugs and drug sundries	4.88	3.65	4.66	10.70	19.67	23.63	25.28	27.23
Eyeglasses and appliances	1.06	.99	1.34	3.09	4.11	5.85	6.58	7.52
Nursing-home care	—	—	.21	1.16	2.63	6.46	7.07	8.70
Expenses for prepayment and administration	.82	.70	1.20	1.89	4.42	6.27	7.26	9.03
Government public health activities	.72	.87	1.16	2.29	2.19	3.41	3.67	4.39
Other health services	.73	.49	.69	3.48	6.91	7.20	8.14	9.64
Research and medical-facilities construction	1.68	.45	1.00	5.52	9.28	16.41	17.32	17.57
Research	—	—	.02	.72	3.21	7.07	7.76	7.98
Construction	1.68	.45	.98	4.80	6.04	9.34	9.56	9.59

Type of expenditure	1968	1969	1970	1971	1972[1]	1973[1]	1974[1]	1975[2]
Total	$264.37	$295.20	$333.57	$368.25	$409.71	$447.31	$484.35	$547.03
Health services and supplies	244.88	274.30	308.81	342.48	380.69	417.10	452.61	513.56
Hospital care	95.31	108.87	124.74	139.03	154.64	169.55	186.06	215.12
Physicians' services	52.78	57.67	64.80	72.05	78.11	84.39	91.12	102.02
Dentists' services	17.30	19.09	21.56	23.42	25.35	28.61	31.58	34.62
Other professional services	5.98	6.32	6.68	7.20	7.72	8.35	8.97	9.69
Drugs and drug sundries	28.84	31.57	34.29	36.39	38.94	42.15	44.75	48.93
Eyeglasses and appliances	8.19	8.49	8.56	8.64	8.88	9.31	10.06	10.62
Nursing-home care	11.60	14.89	18.40	23.34	27.70	31.19	34.69	41.55
Expenses for prepayment and administration	9.53	10.06	10.19	11.48	17.23	20.16	20.96	21.20
Government public health activities	4.92	5.82	6.93	8.10	9.81	10.09	12.22	15.96
Other health services	10.42	11.53	12.65	12.81	12.32	13.30	12.21	13.85
Research and medical-facilities construction	19.49	20.89	24.76	25.77	29.01	30.22	31.73	33.47
Research	8.85	8.72	8.90	8.83	9.73	10.78	11.12	12.69
Construction	10.64	12.18	15.86	16.94	19.29	19.44	20.61	20.77

1. Revised estimates.
2. Preliminary estimates.
3. Based on January 1 data from the Bureau of the Census for total U.S. population (including Armed Forces and Federal civilian employees overseas and the civilian population of outlying areas).

Source: Marjorie Smith Mueller and Robert M. Gibson, "National Health Expenditures, Fiscal Year 1975," *Social Security Bulletin* 39, 2 (February 1976).

Chapter 4

The Federal Government and Health Care

1. THE FEDERAL GOVERNMENT AND HEALTH: OVERVIEW

There is no constitutionally defined role for the federal government in health and therefore such activities have been traditionally reserved to the states. Nevertheless, there has been over the years a gradual development of a federal presence in the field of health. The routes of this still expanding role include:

- the special responsibility for certain population groups, such as merchant seamen, members of the armed forces, veterans, and American Indians;

- responsibilities in the areas of foreign and interstate relationships, such as immigration and quarantine, and the regulation of food and drugs and safety standards;[1]

- grants-in-aid to states, institutions and individuals for a wide variety of activities;

- most recently, sponsorship and financial participation in the health insurance program for the elderly (Medicare).

Many of the federal health-related functions are consolidated in the Department of Health, Education and Welfare (see Section 2, below), Many, however, are among the responsibilities of a variety

---

[1] Much of the regulatory power of the federal government in health, as in other areas, derives from the constitutional power to regulate interstate commerce.

of other departments, agencies, and bureaus, where they generally represent only a part of or are incidental to the main activities of the unit. The more important of these are briefly noted on the following pages.

Executive Office of the President

Office of Management and Budget. This office was organized in 1970, replacing the *Bureau of the Budget.* It is responsible for the preparation, supervision and control of the federal budget and for the overall administration and management of the Executive Branch. This agency thus greatly affects the operation and activities of all federal agencies.

Special Action Office for Drug Abuse Prevention. This office was established in 1971 for overall planning and coordination of federal drug abuse prevention programs.

Department of Agriculture

This department's activities include responsibility for inspection of meat and poultry, and for food and nutrition programs including food stamps, surplus food, and child nutrition.[2]

Department of Defense

The department is responsible for the health and medical care of members of the armed forces through the *Assistant Secretary for Health and Environment.* A complete range of health and medical care programs, institutions and training programs is operated.

Civilian medical care for dependents of servicemen is administered through the CHAMPUS insurance program.[3]

Recent legislation has authorized the establishment of an armed forces medical school.[4]

---

[2] The child nutrition programs include the National School Lunch Program and the National School Breakfast Program, under the National School Lunch Act of 1946, and the Child Nutrition Act of 1966.

[3] Civilian Health and Medical Program of the Uniformed Services, established under the Dependents Medical Care Act of 1956.

[4] Uniformed Services Revitalization Act of 1972.

Department of Housing and Urban Development

This department's programs of assistance for urban development and improvement, especially in low income areas, include provision for the improvement of neighborhood health services. In particular, health-related activities are features of many *Model Cities* programs.[5]

Department of the Interior

This department's *Mining Enforcement and Safety Administration* is responsible for control of health and safety hazards in the mining industry.

Department of Labor

This department's *Occupational Safety and Health Administration* is responsible for the promotion of industrial health and safety and the enforcement of related laws and regulations.[6]

Independent Agencies

There are many federal agencies which are not part of Cabinet departments or the Executive Office. They include a wide variety of administrations, agencies, boards, commissions, councils, etc. Among those with some health-related activities are the following.

ACTION. This agency was established in 1971 to incorporate a number of national volunteer programs, including the Peace Corps, VISTA,[7] the Foster Grandparent Program, and the Retired Senior Volunteer Program.

Appalachian Regional Commission. This commission was created in 1965 by the Appalachian Redevelopment Act. It consists of a

[5] "Model Cities" programs were developed in many urban areas under the Demonstration Cities and Metropolitan Development Act of 1966.

[6] The department's activities in this area were considerably expanded by the Occupational Safety and Health Act of 1970.

[7] Volunteers in Service to America; transferred from the Office of Economic Opportunity.

representative of each of 13 eastern states,[8] a federal co-chairman and a state governor (in rotation) as co-chairman. The purpose of the Commission is to promote the economic, physical and social development of the region. The Commission sponsors a variety of health projects, including community health clinics and manpower training programs.

Community Services Administration.   This agency was established in 1975[9] to replace the Office of Economic Opportunity. It administers the community action programs developed under the Economic Opportunity Act, and a variety of special programs for low income areas. The agency maintains ten regional offices.

Environmental Protection Agency.   This agency was established in 1970 to coordinate and consolidate federal activities in environmental quality control. Its responsibilities include implementation of the Clean Air Act and the Federal Water Pollution Control Act.

General Accounting Office.   The General Accounting Office under the direction of the Comptroller General is an independent agency within the legislative branch. It assists the Congress directly and by carrying out review and auditing of programs and activities authorized by Congress, and makes recommendations designed to make Government operations more efficient and effective. It prescribes the accounting principles and standards to be followed by Federal agencies, and makes determinations as to the legality of actions taken in the use of public funds.

United States Civil Service Commission.   The Commission administers the *Federal Employees Health Benefits Programs*, by contracting with health insurance organizations for health benefit plans.[10]

Veterans Administration.   The Veterans Administration's *Department of Medicine and Surgery* administers the program of medical

---

[8] The Appalachian region, for purposes of the Commission, includes portions of thirteen states: Alabama, Georgia, Kentucky, Maryland, Mississippi, New York, North Carolina, Ohio, Pennsylvania, South Carolina, Tennessee, Virginia, and West Virginia.

[9] Under the Headstart, Economic Opportunity and Community Partnership Act of 1974.

[10] This program was established by the Federal Employees Health Benefits Act of 1959.

services for veterans of the armed forces who have service-related ill-nesses and disabilities, or are medically indigent. Services are rendered through an extensive network of V.A. hospitals, clinics, nursing home and residential units, as well as non-V.A. facilities and practi-tioners. These services are supported by a variety of related man-power training activities including an extensive internship and residency program.

Advisory Groups

There are many advisory groups which have been established for vari-ous levels of government. Of special interest are the following.

Advisory Commission on Intergovernmental Relations. This is a 26-member body established by Congress in 1959 to provide a con-tinuing review of the federal system as it relates to state and local governments. Its membership represents federal, state, and local government and the general public. The Commission publishes annual reports which are of considerable general interest.

Advisory Councils. There are many advisory councils which have been established to advise specific government agencies on various matters including policy, regulations and research grant approval. Ex-amples are the *Health Insurance Benefits Advisory Council* (for Medicare and Medicaid) and the advisory councils to the several institutes of the National Institutes of Health.

Quasi-Official Agencies

There are a number of agencies which, while not formally a part of the federal government, have a special statutory relationship to it. These include the *National Academy of Sciences*[11] (with the National Research Council and the recently organized Institute of Medicine) and the *American National Red Cross.*[12]

---

[11] Established by an Act of Congress in 1863.

[12] Founded by Clara Barton (1882) and chartered under an Act of Congress in 1863.

2. THE DEPARTMENT OF HEALTH, EDUCATION AND WELFARE

Historical Note

The Department of Health, Education and Welfare was created in 1953 by elevating to cabinet status the *Federal Security Agency*, which included most of the federal health, education and social welfare agencies functioning at that time.[13] These include the Public Health Service, Food and Drug Administration, Social Security Administration (with the Children's Bureau), Office of Education and the Office of Vocational Rehabilitation (see Table 4-1).

Public Health Service. The United States Public Health Service was the oldest of HEW's component agencies. It was established by Congress in 1798 as the Marine Hospital Service for the "relief of sick and disabled seamen." This care was financed by monthly contributions of twenty cents from each merchant seaman's wages. The Service was placed in the Treasury Department (where it remained until 1939), and the tax was collected by the Collector of Customs.[14] Gradually, a number of special *marine hospitals* were constructed in principal ports.

In 1878 the Service was authorized by Congress to develop recommendations for uniform quarantine laws and regulations in the states and to carry out investigations related to the cause and control of epidemic disease. Thereafter, the functions of the service steadily increased. Notable dates were the following:

1887—A research program was begun with the establishment of the *Hygienic Laboratory* at the Marine Hospital on Staten Island, New York.

1889—The professional personnel of the Service were organized in a quasi-military *Commissioned Corps* under the Surgeon General.[15]

---

[13] The Federal Security Agency had been created in 1939 to bring together these activities from several departments and agencies.

[14] Later on this tax, the first U.S. compulsory sickness insurance, was discontinued and costs were paid from general revenues.

[15] Initially, members of the Corps were physicians. Membership was broadened by Acts of Congress in 1930 and 1944 to include dentists, sanitary engineers and pharmacists; and dieticians, nurses, physical therapists, sanitarians, scientists and veterinarians.

Table 4-1. Department of Health, Education, and Welfare, 1953*

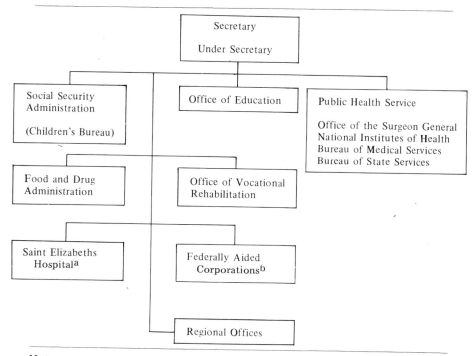

Notes:

[a]A psychiatric hospital for residents of the District of Columbia and persons eligible for care by the Public Health Service or Veterans' Administration.

[b]The federally aided corporations are supported in part by federal funds appropriated in the budget of the Department of Health, Education and Welfare. They are: *American Printing House for the Blind, Columbia Institute for the Deaf* (Kendall School and Gallaudet College), *Howard University*.

*Abbreviated

1893—The Service was given full responsibility for foreign and inter-state quarantine.

1902—The Service was reorganized and renamed the *Public Health and Marine Hospital Service.* It was given responsibility for licensing and regulating the interstate sale of biological products. The Surgeon General was authorized to call an annual conference of state and territorial health officers.

1912—The Service was renamed the United States Public Health Service. In subsequent years, its added responsibilities included the National Leprosarium (Carville, La.), a hospital for the treatment of narcotic addicts (Lexington, Ky.), and a Venereal Disease Control division.

1930—The Hygienic Laboratory was redesignated the *National Institute of Health.*

1935—The Social Security Act's Title VI, administered by the Public Health Service, authorized grants-in-aid to the states for strengthening state and local health departments.

1937—The National Cancer Act created the National Cancer Institute, the first specialty institute in the National Institute of Health.

1939—The Service was transferred from the Treasury Department to the newly established *Federal Security Agency.*

1944—The Public Health Service Act of 1944 (see Section 13) revised substantially and brought together in one statute all existing legislation concerning the Public Health Service.

1946—The Communicable Disease Center was established (Atlanta, Ga.). The Census Bureau's Division of Vital Statistics was transferred to the service as the National Office of Vital Statistics.

1953—The Federal Security Agency became the *Department of Health, Education and Welfare.*

Food and Drug Administration. The Food and Drug Administration was established in the Department of Agriculture in 1927 to administer the several existing acts relating to the quality and safety of food and drugs. It was transferred to the Federal Security Agency in 1940. Its major legislative base was the Food, Drug and Cosmetic Act, originally passed in 1906 (as the Food and Drug Act) and amended many times thereafter.

Social Security Administration. The Social Security Administration (originally the Social Security Board) administered the titles (sections) of the Social Security Act related to Old Age and Survivors Insurance ("social security"), federal aid to state programs for public assistance ("welfare") and unemployment insurance. This agency also included the important *Children's Bureau.*

Children's Bureau. The Children's Bureau was created within the Department of Labor in 1912 to "investigate and report upon . . . all matters pertaining to the welfare of children and child life. . . ." During the next decade it developed an extensive program of studies, research and distribution of educational material relating to the health and welfare of mothers and children.

1921—The Maternity and Infancy Act (Sheppard—Towner Act) provided grants to the states for promotion of maternal and child health work and greatly expanded the scope and activities of the Bureau. Units for child hygiene activities were subsequently established in many states previously without them.

1929—The Maternity and Infancy Act expired and the activities of the Bureau were subsequently curtailed.

1935—Title V of the Social Security Act provided grants-in-aid to the states for maternal and child health, child welfare, and crippled children. The responsibilities of the Bureau were again greatly increased.

1946—The Children's Bureau was transferred from the Department of Labor to the Social Security Administration in the *Federal Security Agency.*

1943
1949—The Bureau administered the *Emergency Maternity and Infant Care Program* for dependents of servicemen.

Office of Education. The Office of Education was established in the Department of the Interior in 1867 to gather statistics and facts and to diffuse information concerning education. Added responsibilities included the administration of grants-in-aid to land grant colleges (1890), and grants to the states for vocational rehabilitation programs (1920–1943) and vocational education programs (1933). The Office became part of the Federal Security Agency in 1939.

Office of Vocational Rehabilitation. The Office of Vocational Rehabilitation was established in 1943 to administer an expanded program of grants to the states for vocational rehabilitation of disabled persons.[16]

Recent Reorganizations of HEW

The Department of Health, Education and Welfare has been reorganized many times since 1953, a process which is still continuing.

[16] Authorized under the Vocational Rehabilitation Act Amendments of 1943.

In 1963, the *Welfare Administration* was established to administer the public assistance and related social service programs. The Children's Bureau was also transferred to this agency, as were the Office of Aging and the Office of Juvenile Delinquency and Youth Development.[17] In 1967, the Welfare Administration and the Vocational Rehabilitation Administration were absorbed into the new *Social and Rehabilitation Service.*

In 1968, the Public Health Service was reorganized with the creation of the *Health Services and Mental Health Administration* (HSMHA) to incorporate most of the traditional functions of the Service. The Service was placed under the direction of the Assistant Secretary for Health and Scientific Affairs with the Surgeon General his principal deputy. A new *Consumer Protection and Environmental Health Services* agency was established, incorporating the Food and Drug Administration. This was shortlived, however, the FDA again becoming a separate agency within the Public Health Service in 1969, and most of the other functions of the Environmental Health Service being transferred in 1970 to the newly created independent *Environmental Protection Agency.*

Another noteworthy reorganization involved the Children's Bureau. In 1969, the Bureau was moved from the Social and Rehabilitation Service to the new Office of Child Development.[18] Its health programs were placed in the new Maternal and Child Health Service (HSMHA) and its social service programs were merged with programs for adults in the Social and Rehabilitation Service. The Bureau retained responsibility for overall coordination of maternal and child health programs, and its original mandate to investigate and report upon matters relating to health and welfare of children. The Office of Child Development also now included the *Head Start* program.[19]

The general organization of HEW in 1972 is shown in Table 4-2. The Health Services and Mental Health Administration is shown in Table 4-3.

Beginning in July 1973, the health agencies of the Department of Health, Education and Welfare were again extensively reorganized. The Health Services and Mental Health Administration was replaced by two new units, the *Health Services Administration* and the *Health*

---

[17] From the Office of the Secretary of HEW.

[18] In the Office of the Secretary of HEW under the Assistant Secretary for Administration.

[19] Transferred from the Office of Economic Opportunity.

Table 4-2. Department of Health, Education, and Welfare, 1972.*

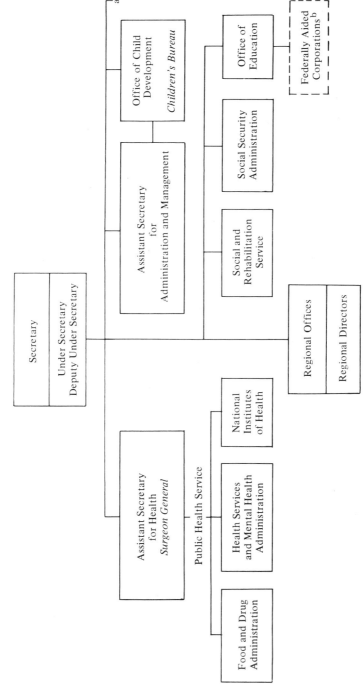

*Abbreviated

[a] Also Assistant Secretaries for: Public Affairs, Community and Field Services, Legislation, and Planning and Evaluation.

[b] American Printing House for the Blind, Gallaudet College, Howard University

Table 4-3. Health Services and Mental Health Administration, 1972

Development	Health Services Delivery

National Center for Health Services
  Research and Development
Health Care Facilities Service
Comprehensive Health Planning Service
Regional Medical Programs Service
Health Maintenance Organization Service
	National Center for Family Planning
	  Services
	Maternal and Child Health Service
	Community Health Service
	Indian Health Service
	Federal Health Programs Service
	National Health Service Corps

Prevention and Consumer Services	**Mental Health**

Center for Disease Control
National Institute of Occupational
  Safety and Health
Bureau of Community Environmental
  Management
	National Institute of Mental Health
	National Institute on Alcohol Abuse
	  and Alcoholism

National Center for Health Statistics

Resources Administration. The Center for Disease Control became a separate agency, and the National Institute of Mental Health became part of a new Alcohol, Drug Abuse and Mental Health Administration. Finally, the functions of the Bureau of Health Manpower Education were transferred from NIH to the new Health Resources Administration.

Additional changes were also made in the Office of the Secretary of HEW. Among these was the establishment of the position of Assistant Secretary of Human Development, whose responsibilities included the Office of Child Development, Office of Youth Development, and the Administration on Aging.[20]

In 1975 the Rehabilitation Services Administration was also transferred to this office from the Social and Rehabilitation Service.

Present Organization of HEW

The Department of Health, Education and Welfare consists of ten operating agencies (Table 4-4). Six are under the rubric of the *Public Health Service*:

Alcohol, Drug Abuse and Mental Health Administration
Center for Disease Control

---

[20] The Administration on Aging was transferred from the Social and Rehabilitation Service subsequent to provisions of the 1973 amendments of the Older Americans Act.

Table 4-4. Department of Health, Education and Welfare, 1976.*

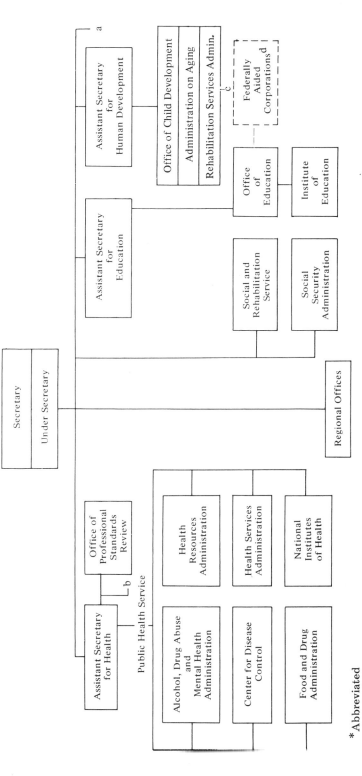

*Abbreviated

[a] Also Assistant Secretaries for Public Affairs, Legislation, Planning and Evaluation, Administration and Management, and a Comptroller

[b] Also: Office of International Health, Office of Population Affairs, Office of Nursing Home Affairs

[c] Also: Office of Youth Development, Office for Handicapped Individuals, Office of Native American Programs, Office of Rural Development

[d] American Printing House for the Blind, Gallaudet College, Howard University

Food and Drug Administration
Health Resources Administration
Health Services Administration
National Institutes of Health

The other four agencies are:

Social Security Administration
Social and Rehabilitation Service
Office of Education[21]
National Institute of Education[21]

Additional agencies, under the rubric of the Office of Human Development (Assistant Secretary for Human Development) include the Administration on Aging and the Rehabilitation Services Administration.

Public Health Service

The Public Health Service is completely under the direction of the Assistant Secretary for Health. No specific functions have been assigned to the Surgeon General, and this position is now vacant.[22] Among the administrative units of the Assistant Secretary's office is the *Office of Professional Standards Review* which has the responsibility for professional standards review organization (PSRO) activities.

Alcohol, Drug Abuse and Mental Health Administration. This agency was established in 1973 and incorporated the following three agencies:

National Institute on Alcohol Abuse and Alcoholism—responsible for programs directed toward the problems of alcohol abuse.

National Institute on Drug Abuse—administers programs directed to the problems of drug abuse.

National Institute of Mental Health—This agency was established in 1946 as the second specialty institute of the Public Health Service. It was separated from the National Institutes of Health as a separate

---

[21] The Office of Education and the National Institute of Education make up the *Division of Education*. The Institute was established under the Education Amendments of 1972.

[22] An Acting Surgeon General continues to carry out certain statutory functions, including administrative responsibilities related to the Commissioned Corps.

bureau in 1967, and in 1968 was incorporated into the new Health Services and Mental Health Administration. It administers programs of research, service development and training in mental health, including support of community health centers.

Center for Disease Control (Atlanta). This is the former Communicable Disease Center, which was renamed in 1970 when its functions were broadened to include, in addition to its traditional activities related to infectious disease, other preventable conditions including malnutrition.

The Center conducts and supports programs for prevention and control of disease and provides consultation and assistance to state and local health departments and other countries, including extensive epidemiological services. It is also responsible for foreign quarantine activities.

Under the 1973 Public Health Service reorganization, the Center incorporated the National Institute of Occupational Safety and Health.[23] including the Appalachian Laboratory of Occupational Respiratory Disease. It also took over from the former Bureau of Community Environmental Management the functions related to lead poisoning prevention and rat control.

Food and Drug Administration. This agency is responsible for determining the safety of foods, drugs, cosmetics, and therapeutic devices; for proper labeling and product information; and approval of all new drugs for marketing. The 1962 Kefauver-Harris amendments to the Pure Food, Drug and Cosmetics Act require in addition that the FDA consider efficacy as well as safety in making decisions regarding drugs and therapeutic devices.

Health Resources Administration. This agency is concerned with the planning, development and distribution of health resources, including manpower training.

National Center for Health Statistics. The Center collects and reports the official U.S. vital statistics. It carries out a continuing program of studies, data evaluation and methods research in health and vital statistics. These include special continuing surveys, including:

---

[23] The National Institute of Occupational Safety and Health conducts research and studies and develops standards.

- *The Health Interview Survey*—a national household interview study of illness, disability, and health services utilization.[24]
- *The Health and Nutrition Examination Survey*—a program of examination and testing of national population samples.
- *The Hospital Discharge Survey*—a survey of patient utilization of short stay hospitals.
- *The Master Facility Inventory Survey*—periodically surveys all U.S. health facilities.
- *The Ambulatory Medical Care Survey*—was begun in 1973. Data is collected from a sample of practicing physicians.

The Center is also participating in and provides some grant support for the development of a federal-state-local *Cooperative Health Statistics System.*

National Center for Health Services Research. The Center conducts and supports research and demonstration projects related to the financing, organization and delivery of health care. Special emphasis has been given to the areas of cost, quality and new types of health manpower. The Center divisions are:

- Division of Health Services Research Strategy
- Division of Health Services Evaluation
- Division of Long Term Care
- Division of Health Services Research and Analysis
- Division of Health Services Quality Research
- Division of Health Systems Design and Development
- Division of Health Care Information Systems and Technology.

Bureau of Health Planning and Resources Development.[25] This Bureau administers the program of support for state and area health planning and development agencies and activities; and the Hill-Burton program of loans and grants for the construction and modernization of health facilities. Its divisions are:

- Division of Agency Development
- Division of Planning Methods Technology
- Division of Facilities Development
- Division of Regulatory Activities

[24] This was the first system for the regular collection of health related data by the Public Health Service. It was developed under the National Health Survey Act of 1956.

[25] Primarily responsible for implementing the provisions of the National Health Planning and Resources Development Act of 1974.

Bureau of Health Manpower. The health manpower development activities of the Public Health Service, including grant support for education and training, are carried out by this Bureau through the following divisions:

- Division of Medicine
- Division of Nursing
- Division of Dentistry
- Division of Associated Health Professions

Health Services Administration. This agency is concerned with the support of programs related to health services delivery.

Indian Health Service—administers the system of hospitals and health centers which provides health services to American Indians and native Alaskans.

Bureau of Medical Services—administers the Public Health Service hospitals and clinics,[26] and provides work related health services for federal employees. The Division of Emergency Health Services supports emergency medical care systems development and provides medical assistance in disasters. Activities related to the development of health maintenance organizations were transferred from the Bureau of Community Health Services in 1975.

Bureau of Community Health Services—administers programs related to maternal and child health,[27] family planning, comprehensive health centers, (neighborhood health centers), and migrant health. It also includes the *National Health Service Corps*, a program for deployment of Public Health Service personnel, including physicians, to areas of particular need.

Bureau of Quality Assurance—promotes and supports activities related to standards and evaluation of health care services.[28] Responsibilities include implementation of the PSRO program.

[26] Eight general hospitals and a hospital for leprosy patients in Carvill, Louisiana. (In 1948, there were 24 hospitals. Many have since been closed or turned over to local communities.)

[27] Under Title V of the Social Security Act.

[28] Including the End Stage Renal Disease Program (ERDP) for the renal dialysis and transplants under Medicare.

National Institute of Health. This agency, nominally with the Public Health Service, includes the National Library of Medicine,[29] the Fogarty International Center for the Advanced Study of Health Sciences, and eleven *research institutes* which carry out and support programs of basic and clinical research. They are:

- National Institute on Aging
- National Cancer Institute
- National Heart and Lung Institute
- National Institute of Dental Research
- National Institute of Neurological Disease and Stroke
- National Institute of Arthritis, Metabolism and Digestive Diseases
- National Institute of Allergy and Infectious Diseases
- National Institute of Child Health and Human Development
- National Institute of General Medical Sciences
- National Eye Institute
- National Institute of Environmental Health Sciences

Non-PHS Agencies

Social Security Administration. This agency is responsible for the Old Age, Survivors, and Disability Insurance Program (OASDI) and for administering most of the program of Health Insurance for the Aged (Medicare). It administers the recently established program of Supplemental Security Income for the Aged, Blind and Disabled.[30] It is also responsible for review and authorization of claims for black-lung benefits under the Federal Coal Mine Health and Safety Act of 1969. The *Office of Research and Statistics* collects and analyzes data concerning health costs and expenditures and publishes many reports.

The SSA divisions are:

- Bureau of Data Processing
- Bureau of Disability Insurance
- Bureau of District Office Operations
- Bureau of Health Insurance
- Bureau of Hearings and Appeals
- Bureau of Retirement and Survivors Insurance

---

[29] The Library carries on a wide variety of informational activities, including publication of the *Index Medicus*, and development and operation of the Medical Literature and Analysis Retrieval System (MEDLARS).

[30] Under provisions of the Social Security Amendments of 1972.

- Bureau of Supplemental Security Income of the Aged, Blind and Disabled.

Social and Rehabilitation Service. This agency administers programs of grants to the states for:

- Public assistance to families with dependent children (Aid to Families with Dependent Children, AFDC).
- Medical assistance (Medicaid).
- Social services under the AFDC program including foster care, day care, and family planning services.
- Social services for aged, blind, and disabled adults.

The SRS divisions are:

- Assistance Payments Administration
- Community Services Administration
- Medical Services Administration

The *Rehabilitation Services Administration* was transferred to the Office of Human Development in 1975.[31] This Services is responsible for programs related to rehabilitation of the disabled particularly vocational rehabilitation.

Office of Education. The Office has retained its original statutory mandate to gather statistics and diffuse information concerning education. In addition, it administers many grant programs related to elementary, secondary and higher education. The Office also sets standards and criteria for the recognition, for purposes of federal funding, of voluntary agencies which accredit educational institutions and programs (including those engaged in *health manpower education and training*).

National Institute of Education. The Institute was established in 1972 to coordinate research and development programs in education.

In addition to the agencies described above, the important *Administration on Aging* should be noted. It is located in the Office of Human Development, and administers programs relating to problems of the aged under provisions of the Older Americans Act.

[31] Under the Rehabilitation Act Amendments of 1974.

HEW Regional Offices

There are ten regional offices[32] of the Department of Health, Education and Welfare, each with a regional director. Their staffs work cooperatively with state and local government and community agencies in carrying out departmental programs. Their responsibilities include the review and approval of grant applications.

References

United States Government Manual, official handbook of the Federal Government, published annually by the office of the Federal Register (General Services Administration).

Annual reports of the Department of Health, Education and Welfare, U.S. Government Printing Office, 1953–1971.

3. INTRODUCTION TO HEALTH LEGISLATION

The many activities of the federal government in health are authorized by the passage of laws, or statutes, by the Congress.

The Enactment of Laws[33]

Proposed legislation, called a *bill*,[34] is introduced in the Senate or House of Representatives by a congressional sponsor.[35] It is assigned a sequential number (i.e., HR-1, S-3) and referred to the appropriate committee for study. Public *hearings* are often held, after which the bill may be amended or entirely redrafted, sometimes in combination with other bills addressed to the same issue. Ultimately, if it is approved, the bill is discharged from the committee with a favorable report and is then placed on the legislative calendar for floor action. (A committee does not act on every bill referred to it and there is no time limit within which it must report out a bill.)

---

[32] The offices are: I Boston, II New York, III Philadelphia, IV Atlanta, V Chicago, VI Dallas, VII Kansas City, Mo., VIII Denver, IX San Francisco, X Seattle.

[33] This is a general outline of a very complex process.

[34] Occasionally, legislation is introduced as a *resolution* which has essentially the same practical significance as a bill.

[35] Legislation may be drafted by legislators and their staffs, by various levels of the Executive Branch, or by private citizens or groups. A bill may have a number of Congressional sponsors, up to 25 in the House and unlimited in the Senate.

If passed by the Senate or House (with or without amendments from the floor), the bill is sent to the other chamber where essentially the same process of committee referral, reporting, and floor debate takes place.

If there is substantial disagreement between the two houses on a bill which has been passed by both, *Conference Committees* will be formed from among the members of the committees which reported the bill. If an agreement is arrived at, a *conference report* is made which is then voted on as a whole, without amendment, by each house. If passed by both houses it is sent to the President for approval. When signed by him, the bill becomes a law or *statute.*

Any legislation which has not been finally passed by both the Senate and House of Representatives by the end of a Congress[36] is dead and must be re-introduced in the next Congress if it is to be again considered. (Only a minority of the many bills introduced in each legislative session become a law.)

The law is then numbered sequentially and by number of the Congress; for example, Public Law 89-97 (PL 89-97) means the 97th law passed by the 89th Congress.[37] The law is printed in pamphlet form known as a *slip law;* later it is published in the *Statutes at Large* and ultimately incorporated into the *United States Code.*

The formal title, which is an integral part of the law, takes the form "An Act to . . ." and may be quite detailed. Often a *short title* is also specified. Frequently, however, a law comes to be known by the names of its chief Congressional sponsors. For example, PL79-725 is formally entitled "An Act to amend the Public Health Service Act to authorize grants to the states for surveying their hospital and public health centers and for planning construction of additional facilities, and to authorize grants to assist in such construction." Its short title is the "Hospital Survey and Construction Act." However, it is generally known as the "Hill-Burton Act" after its sponsors, Senators Lister Hill and Harold Burton.

Occasionally a specific section of an Act may be given a specific short title. For example, Title (section) I of PL 92-157 is the *Comprehensive Health Manpower Training Act of 1971.*

Rarely, a law will retain as its popular name its original bill num-

---

[36] The two annual sessions spanning the term of office of members of the House of Representatives are known as a Congress. For example, the 92nd Congress extended from Janury 1971 to December 1972.

[37] There is also a series of *Private Laws* relating to private individuals or claims against the government.

ber, notably the *Social Security Amendments of 1972,* which were for a time widely referred to as "HR-1." Sometimes a part of a law will acquire a popular name. For example, the Professional Standards Review Organizations (PSRO) section of the Social Security Amendments of 1972 is often called the "Bennett Amendment" after Senator Wallace Bennett, who amended the original bill with these provisions.

Much legislation is "authorizing" legislation which establishes or continues programs and authorizes funding for them. *Appropriations bills* actually provide the funds. Often, less is appropriated than has been authorized to be appropriated. Furthermore, the Executive branch may not elect to spend all the funds appropriated for a particular purpose if these were more than requested or if it does not wish to implement a particular program.

The actual power of the President to "impound" funds appropriated by Congress has been a controversial Constitutional question between the Legislative and Executive branches of the government. This has been settled for practical purposes by the *Impoundment Control Act of 1974* whereby the President may temporarily impound funds but must ask the Congress to *rescind* specified appropriations if he wishes not to spend the funds at all.

Regulations

Many of the details of the various laws are left to be spelled out in *regulations* prescribed by the various administrative agencies of the Executive Branch. As these are made, they are published in the *Federal Register*, taking effect 30 days thereafter.[38] These regulations are then incorporated in the *Code of Federal Regulations* and have the force of law.

Congressional Committees

There are 18 standing committees in the Senate and 22 in the House of Representatives, as well as a number of special and joint committees. Many committees may be involved in the various matters relating to health, but those of particular importance are:

- House Ways and Means Committee:[39] Subcommittee on Health

---

[38] Often these are published as proposed regulations, which are then revised as final regulations after comments have been received from interested parties.

[39] Has jurisdiction over the Social Security laws (except programs supported from general revenues). This is due to the Constitutional provision that laws to raise revenue must originate in the House; such (tax) measures are assigned to this committee.

- Senate Finance Committee: Subcommittee on Health
- House Interstate and Foreign Commerce Committee: Subcommittee on Health and the Environment
- Senate Labor and Public Welfare Committee: Subcommittee on Health
- House Appropriations Committee: Subcommittee for Labor, and Health, Education and Welfare
- Senate Appropriations Committee: Subcommittee for Labor, and Health, Education and Welfare

Other important committees are:

- House and Senate Budget Committees
- House Rules Committee[40]
- Senate Special Committee on Aging

Grants-in-Aid

Many of the funds distributed to the states and localities under federal legislation are made available by the mechanism of *grants-in-aid*. These grants are authorized in the various federal laws for stated purposes and are given to the states and to local organizations, agencies and individuals, under certain conditions and in accordance with certain regulations.

Formula grants—Funds are allotted by a formula which takes into consideration such factors as state population, per capita income, and the extent of health problems.

Matching grants—Funds must be matched up to a specified percentage by the state, agency, or institution receiving the grant. For example, for certain construction grants under the Hill-Burton program: "The Federal share . . . may not exceed 66-2/3 percent."

Research grants—Funds are granted competitively to individuals, agencies, and institutions to carry out specific research work outlined in research proposals submitted by the applicants.[41]

Training grants—Funds are granted competitively to institutions

[40] Determines the order in which bills are considered by the House and the rules under which they are debated.

[41] In recent years federal agencies have made considerable use of the *contract* mechanism for funding health related research, studies and other activities. "Requests for proposals" (RFP's) are circulated by the funding agency to institutions, agencies and individuals active in the area of the proposed work

engaged in certain health manpower training activities. These may include student stipends.

Capitation grants—Funds are allotted to educational institutions by formulas related to student enrollment.

"Categorical grants" are made for relatively narrowly defined categories of problems, i.e., entities such as chronic disease, venereal disease.

"Block grants" are for more broadly defined purposes, such as public health services in general, and permit more discretion in use of the funds.

Grants-in-aid to the states are usually made from allotments among the states in accordance with the specified formula. These grants also carry such requirements as the submission of a *state plan* concerning the problem or purpose in question, assignment of the responsibility for administration of the plan to a *single state agency* and conformation to guidelines and standards regarding use of the funds. They are typically formula grants, and generally have matching requirements.

Programs of grants-in-aid are usually authorized for stipulated periods of time only, usually two to five years; these authorizations must be renewed periodically if programs are to continue. Thus, at any point in time, several of these will be in various stages of the legislative process, for continuation and amendment.[42]

The concept of *revenue sharing* has been advocated as a more appropriate mechanism for financial aid to the states than the relatively categorical approach of the grant-in-aid programs. The first revenue sharing legislation was passed in 1972.[43] Whether such a mechanism should ultimately largely replace the grant-in-aid structure, especially in the health field, has been a subject of some controversy.

---

[42] One exception is the research and training grants of The National Institutes of Health which have no statutory time limit, though subject to the usual appropriations bills.

[43] The State and Local Fiscal Assistance Act of 1972. Funds are allocated to state governments with relatively few restrictions. Local governments must use their funds for "priority expenditures": necessary capital expenditures, and operating expenses in the areas of public safety, environmental protection, public transportation, health, recreation, libraries, social service for the poor and aged, and financial administration.

Specific Health Legislation

The following sections summarize the principal federal legislation related to health care. They do not attempt to deal with the complex political, social, and economic background of this body of legislation, nor with its implementation and impact. They are designed to provide a base from which to address these issues.

The material is presented in such a way as to give a general sense of the historical development of these laws which have had and will continue to have a profound effect on the health care scene.

The Social Security Act, and the Public Health Service Act are described in particular detail, as they have been the vehicles for such important health-related programs as Medicare and Medicaid and the Hill-Burton, comprehensive health planning and health manpower programs.

References

How Our Laws Are Made, Charles I. Zinn. House of Representatives Document No. 93-377, 1974.

Guide to the Congress. (Washington, D.C.: Congressional Quarterly, 1971).

Selected Readings

The following books illustrate well the workings of the legislative process:

The Dance of Legislation, Eric Redman (New York: Simon and Schuster, 1973).

Politics, Science and Dread Disease, Stephen P. Strickland (Cambridge, Massachusetts: Harvard University Press, 1972).

A Sacred Trust, Richard Harris (New York: New America Library, 1966). History of the Medicare legislation.

NOTE: There are many official *government document depositories*, containing selected documents, in public and university libraries throughout the country. Some of these are *regional depositories* which receive copies of most documents published by the Government Printing Office.

4. THE SOCIAL SECURITY ACT

"An Act to provide for the general welfare by establishing a system of federal old age benefits, and by enabling the several States to make more adequate provision for aged persons, blind persons, dependent and crippled children, maternal and child welfare, public health, and the administration of their unemployment compensation laws; to establish a Social Security Board: to raise revenue; and for other purposes."

The Social Security Act of 1935 was a landmark piece of legislation which was developed and passed during the Great Depression. It represented the first major entrance of the federal government into the area of social insurance and it greatly and significantly expanded federal grant-in-aid assistance to the states. It has formed the base for important federal programs in health including, most recently, Medicare and Medicaid.

The original legislation consisted of eleven Titles (divisions). (See Appendix C). In summary, these:

- Established the "Social Security" program of old age benefits. (Title I)
- Provided for federal financial assistance to the states' public assistance ("welfare") programs for the needy elderly, dependent children and the blind. (Titles I, IV, X)
- Provided fiscal incentives for the establishment of state unemployment funds. (Title III)
- Established financial assistance for maternal and child health and child welfare services (Title V) and greatly increased such assistance for state and local public health programs (Title VI).[44]

Amendments

In the ensuing years, there have been many *amendments* to the original Social Security Act, enlarging gradually the scope of its provisions.

In 1939 benefits for dependents and survivors were added to the old age program and in 1956 a federal program of disability benefits was added. The program was now known as Old Age, Survivors and Disability Insurance (OASDI).

In 1950 the program of federal aid to state public assistance programs was extended to disabled persons (Title XIV). (Federal participation in state payments to providers of medical services [vendor payments] to persons on public assistance was also added.) The "federally aided public assistance categories" established under the Act (initially and by amendment) were now:

---

[44] The Title VI provisions were subsequently incorporated into the Public Health Service Act (1944).

- Old Age Assistance (OAA)
- Aid to Families with Dependent Children (AFDC)
- Aid to the Blind (AB)
- Aid to the Permanently and Totally Disabled (APTD)

Among subsequent legislation were the following important health-related amendments:

The Kerr-Mills Act (1960). The Social Security Amendments of 1960 ("Kerr-Mills" Act) established a program providing payments for medical care for needy elderly persons not receiving public assistance ("medically indigent aged"). This was the forerunner of the Medicaid Program.

1963 Maternal and Child Health Provisions. The 1963 amendments (Maternal and Child Health and Mental Retardation Planning Amendments) added to Title V authorization for special project grants for comprehensive programs of maternity and infant care.

Medicare and Medicaid (1965). The Social Security amendments of 1965 added two new sections to the Act: Title XVIII, *Health Insurance for the Aged*, and Title XIX, *Grants to the States for Medical Assistance Payments*; these came to be known as "Medicare" and "Medicaid". Also, special project grants for comprehensive programs for *children and youth* were added to Title V.

Social Security Amendments of 1967. A number of adjustments were made in the Medicare and Medicaid programs (including provisions for limitation of federal participation in the latter) and in the Title V programs.

Social Security Amendments of 1972 ("H.R.-1"). Among the many important provisions in these amendments were many related to the Medicare and Medicaid programs. These included the bringing of many disabled persons under Medicare, and the establishment of Professional Standard Review Organizations (PSRO's).

These amendments are described in more detail in the following pages.

Selected Readings

The Development of the Social Security Act: A Memorandum on the History of the Committee on Economic Security and Drafting and Legislative History of the Social Security Act. Edwin E. Witte, (Madison: University of Wisconsin Press, 1963).

Social Security Programs in the United States, U.S. Department of Health, Education and Welfare, Social Security Administration. This is an excellent summary of programs related to the Social Security Act. It is revised periodically, following major amendments.

Basic Readings in Social Security, U.S. Department of Health, Education and Welfare, Social Security Administration, Office of Research and Statistics, 1973. A good bibliography on the subject of Social Security.

5. SOCIAL SECURITY AMENDMENTS OF 1960 "KERR-MILLS" ACT

The most important provisions of the 1960 amendments were those related to medical services for the aged, provisions which were passed after extensive congressional debate concerning health insurance for the aged.

Title I of the Social Security Act was amended to read *Grants to the States for Old Age Assistance and Medical Assistance for the Aged:*

". . . .for the purpose of enabling each state to furnish medical assistance on behalf of aged individuals who are not recipients of old age assistance but whose income and resources are insufficient to meet the costs of necessary medical services. . . ."

This established a new program of *medical assistance for the aged* (MAA) providing for federal aid to the states for payments for medical care for "medically indigent" persons age 65 and over. This became known as the Kerr-Mills program.

Participation by the states was optional. Under the program:

- A broad range of medical services could be made available with the stipulation that at least *some institutional* and *some non-institutional* care be available to the recipients.
- No lien could be made on a recipient's property during his lifetime (and lifetime of spouse).
- No duration of residence requirement could be made for any person residing in the state.
- Federal participation to be 50-80 percent of program costs, according to per capita income in the state.
- Federal sharing was excluded for payments for persons in non-medical institutions and persons in tuberculosis and mental hospitals.

6. MATERNAL AND CHILD HEALTH AND MENTAL RETARDATION PLANNING AMENDMENTS OF 1963

"An Act to amend the Social Security Act to assist States and communities in preventing and combating mental retardation through expansion and improvement of the maternal and child health and crippled children's programs, through provision of prenatal, maternity, and infant care for individuals with conditions associated with childbearing which may lead to mental retardation, and through planning for comprehensive action to combat mental retardation, and for other purposes."

The 1963 Social Security Amendments made several additions to Title V:

- Increased funds were authorized for Maternal and Child Health and Crippled Children's Services.
- Special Project Grants for Maternity and Infant Care—"In order to help reduce the incidence of mental retardation caused by complications associated with childbearing" there were authorized to state health agencies and, with the consent of such agency, to any local health agency grants for "projects for the provision of necessary health care to prospective mothers (including, after childbirth, health care to mothers and their infants) who have or are likely to have conditions associated with childbearing which increase the hazards to the health of the mothers or their infants . . . and whom the state or local health agency determines will not receive necessary health care because they are from low income families or for other reasons beyond their control." Federal participation: 75 percent of costs.
- Grants were also authorized for *research projects* relating to maternal and child health services and crippled children's services.

A new title was also added to the Social Security Act: Title XVII, *Grants for Planning Comprehensive Action to Combat Mental Retardation.*

Grants were authorized to assist the states to plan for comprehensive state and community action to combat mental retardation.[45] Federal participation: 75 percent of costs.

[45] This provision for planning grants has since expired.

7. SOCIAL SECURITY AMENDMENTS OF 1965*

"An Act to provide a hospital insurance program for the aged under the Social Security Act with a supplementary medical benefits program and an expanded program of medical assistance, to increase benefits under the Old-Age, Survivors, and Disability Insurance System, to improve the Federal-State public assistance programs, and for other purposes."

The Social Security amendments of 1965 established the national program of health insurance for the aged now known as "Medicare."[46] It was the culmination of many years of national and Congressional debate and is of great historic importance. The amendments also included provisions for expansion of the Kerr-Mills medical assistance program to groups other than the elderly—a program now known as "Medicaid." Significant additions were made to Title V, and changes were also made in the OASDI and Public Assistance titles of the Social Security Act.

Health Insurance for the Aged (Medicare)

Title XVIII, *Health Insurance for the Aged*, was added to the Social Security Act. Because of the importance of this legislation, a relatively extensive summary of the original provisions is set forth below.

Part A: Hospital Insurance Benefits. This insurance program provides basic protection against the costs of hospital and related post-hospital services. Benefits include:

- *Inpatient hospital* services up to 90 days during any spell of illness and psychiatric inpatient services up to 190 days lifetime.
- Post-hospital *extended care* services up to 100 days during any spell of illness.
- Post-hospital *home health* services up to 100 visits in a one-year period.
- Hospital outpatient *diagnostic* services.

Part B: Supplemental Medical Insurance Benefits. This is a voluntary insurance program financed from premium payments by enrollees and contributions from federal funds. Benefits include:

---

*PL 89-97.

[46] This term was originally applied to the program for medical care for servicemen's dependents under the Dependents Medical Care Act (1956). It is now universally applied to this program of health insurance for the aged.

- *Physicians' services*, and services related to a physician's professional services
- *Home health* services

Because of the importance of this legislation, a relatively extensive summary of the original provisions is set forth in Appendix D.

Federal-State Medical Assistance Program (Medicaid)

Title XIX, *Grants to the States for Medical Assistance Programs*, was added to the Social Security Act.

This title established a single program of medical assistance for public assistance recipients, and extended eligibility to medically indigent persons not on welfare. It is a federal-state matching grant program.

Under the program, states were to provide at least some of each of five basic services:

- Inpatient hospital services
- Outpatient hospital services
- Other laboratory and X-ray services
- Skilled nursing home services
- Physicians' services

Additional services could also be made available by the states. The federal share of the program's costs is 53–80 percent, according to a state's per capita income.

For a more detailed summary of this title, see Appendix E.

Maternal and Child Health Services

There were a number of amendments to Title V. (See Appendix F.) Most notable was the provision for special project grants for comprehensive services for *children and youth*. These children and youth (C&Y) projects and the maternal and infant care (M&I) projects developed under the 1963 amendments have formed the core services of many neighborhood health centers.

8. SOCIAL SECURITY AMENDMENTS, 1966-1971

During 1966 and 1967 there were several short amendments to the Medicare section of the Social Security Act, providing for extension of the initial and first general enrollment periods, and adjusting the reimbursement formula for proprietary extended care facilities.

Social Security Amendments of 1967

These extensive amendments included a number of changes and adjustments in the Medicare and Medicaid programs:

Medicare-Amendments

- Provision for direct payment to the patient for physicians' services on the basis of an *itemized bill*—not necessarily a receipted (paid) bill.
- Elimination of the requirement that a physician *certify* to the medical necessity of admissions to general hospitals and of outpatient hospital services; (the requirement for periodic certification after admission remains).
- Inclusion under Part B of the services of *podiatrists* for non-routine foot care.
- Transfer of hospital *outpatient diagnostic services* from Part A to Part B.
- Provision for the payment of *full reasonable charges for radiologists' and pathologists' services* to inpatients; (deductible and co-insurance no longer applicable to these services).
- Provision for purchase of durable medical equipment for use in the home.
- Inclusion of outpatient *physical therapy* under Part B.
- Provision for payment under Part B for *diagnostic X-rays* taken in a patient's home or nursing home.
- Addition of a *lifetime reserve of 60 days* of coverage for inpatient hospital care; (coinsurance of one-half the inpatient deductible).
- Transfer of the responsibilities of the National Medical Review Committee (members not yet appointed) to the Health Insurance Benefits Advisory Council, which is enlarged to 19 members.

Medicaid Amendments

- Provision for *limitation of federal participation* in medical assistance payments to families whose income does not exceed 133 percent of the income limit for AFDC payments in any state.

- For the medically indigent, the states may select the "basic five" services or seven out of the first 14 of the services listed under the original legislation. The states must continue to provide the "basic five" services for public assistance recipients.
- Requirement, as of July 1969, that the states provide health screening services for Medicaid eligible children and such corrective measures as provided in regulations.
- If nursing home or hospital services are selected, physicians' services in these institutions are also to be included.
- Establishment of an *Advisory Council on Medical Assistance*, consisting of 21 persons, to advise the Secretary in matters of administration of the program.
- Provision that persons covered under medical assistance will have free choice of qualified medical facilities and practitioners.
- Requirements that skilled nursing homes providing services under the medical assistance program meet the requirements for state licensure, and meet standards similar to those applicable to extended care facilities; that their administration be licensed; and that there be a program of regular medical review of care furnished.

Maternal and Child Health Amendments[47]

- Revised Title V to consolidate all its programs for maternal and child health and crippled children under one authorization
- Continued provisions for special projects (40 percent of appropriated funds) for maternal and infant care and for health of school and pre-school children ["children and youth projects"] and added authorization for special projects for dental health of children.
- Made special provision for funding of family planning services[48]
- As of June 30, 1972, 90 percent of appropriated funds to be for formula grants to the states (under which the special projects may be continued by the states) and 10 percent for training and research projects[49]
- Continued and expanded provisions for training of personnel, and added authorization for research projects related to maternal and child health and crippled children's services
- Transferred authorization for child welfare services to Title IV

A provision was also included (Title XI) for federal participation

[47] Child Health Act of 1967

[48] Not less than six percent of funds appropriated for maternal and child health services, maternity and infant care projects, and related research projects.

[49] Provision postponed by subsequent amendments to June 30, 1974.

in payment for services in *intermediate care* facilities[50] for public assistance recipients.

In 1969, a rider was added to an unrelated bill (PL 91-55) providing for additional modifications of the Medicaid program:

- Extension to July 1, 1977 of the deadline for states to establish comprehensive medical assistance programs.
- The states are permitted to reduce some medical services previously available under their medical assistance programs (but prohibiting reduction of cash payments to public assistance recipients).

An additional amendment in 1971 (PL 92-223) broadened the intermediate care facilities provisions to include, optionally, Medicaid recipients other than those on public assistance.

9. SOCIAL SECURITY AMENDMENTS OF 1972*

"An Act to amend the Social Security Act, and for other purposes."

The Social Security Amendments of 1972 made important changes in the Social Security Act, including extensive amendments of the Medicare and Medicaid provisions.

Title 1. Provisions Relating to Old Age, Survivors and Disability Insurance

This title makes a number of adjustments in OASDI provisions for various categories of beneficiaries.

Title II. Provisions Relating to Medicare, Medicaid and Maternal and Child Health

This title incorporates a large number of amendments (97 separate sections) affecting Medicare and Medicaid, many addressed to the control of costs, many making significant changes. Notable among the provisions are the following:[51]

Health Insurance for the Disabled. Persons who have received

---

[50] An institution providing a level of care beyond room and board, but not of a degree required of a skilled nursing home.

*PL 92-603.

[51] Briefly summarized.

cash benefits under the disability insurance provisions of the Social Security Act for at least 24 months will be eligible for medical benefits under Title XVIII of the Social Security Act (which will now read *Health Insurance for the Aged and Disabled*).

Part B. Premiums, Deductibles and Automatic Enrollment. Part B premiums will not be increased more than the most recent percentage increase in social security cash benefits. Beneficiaries will be automatically enrolled upon entitlement with provision made for those who wish to decline enrollment. The annual deductible is increased to $60.

Cost Sharing Under Medicaid. (1) The states must charge an income-related enrollment fee to medically indigent persons included under Medicaid programs, and may charge nominal deductibles and co-payments; (2) The states may charge public assistance recipients nominal deductibles and co-payments for other than the basic mandated services.

Deferred Loss of Medicaid Due to Increased Earnings. Families who lose Medicaid eligibility because of increased earnings will remain covered for four months.

Limitation of Payments for Unnecessary Capital Expenditures. Payment will not be made for capital expenditures which have been disapproved by State or local planning agencies.

Experiments and Demonstrations Related to Increased Economy and Efficiency of Health Services. Grants and contracts are authorized for studies, experiments and demonstrations related to prospective reimbursement; the three-day hospitalization requirement for skilled nursing home admission; ambulatory surgical centers, intermediate care facilities; home health and day care services; payment for services of physician's assistants and nurse practitioners; and use of clinical psychologists.

Health Maintenance Organizations. Single annual per capita payments may be made to health maintenance organizations[52] for Part A and Part B services provided to or arranged for Medicare beneficiaries. Such organizations must provide care to a group of enrollees

[52] The definition of such organizations includes (1) provision, either directly or through arrangements, of services to enrolled individuals on the basis of a predetermined periodic rate regardless of the frequency or extent of services and (2) provision of services primarily through such organization's physicians or under arrangements with groups of physicians (in group or individual practice) which are reimbursed on the basis of an aggregate fixed sum or per capita basis.

of whom at least one half are not Medicare beneficiaries. Up to 20 percent of any savings made by a health maintenance organization relative to the per capita annual costs of services to non-HMO enrollees will be divided equally between the organization and the Medicare trust funds.

Payment of Teaching Physicians.   Payment under Part B for services of physicians in hospital teaching programs will generally be made on a cost basis only except for bona fide private patients. Payment for donated services of such physicians will be made to a fund designated for charitable or educational purposes.

Advance Approval of Skilled Nursing Facility and Home Health Benefits.   Minimum periods of presumed eligibility for post-hospital services may be established by the Secretary.

Elimination of Requirement of Progressively More Comprehensive Medicaid Programs.   The Title IX section requiring that the states progress toward the provision of comprehensive Medicaid services by July 1, 1977 is repealed.

Level of State Medicaid Funding.   The Title IX section prohibiting a state from reducing its aggregate payments for Medicaid services is repealed.

Payments to States for Claims and Information Systems.   Matching funds may be paid to the states for development and installation of claims processing and information retrieval systems (90 percent of costs) and, under certain conditions, for their operation (75 percent of costs).

Utilization Review Under Medicaid and Child Health Programs. Hospitals and skilled nursing facilities participating in Medicaid or child health programs must, with some exceptions, use the same utilization review committees as are used under the Medicare program.

Validation of Joint Commission on Accreditation of Hospitals Surveys.   Arrangements are authorized for the state Medicare certifying agencies to survey, by sampling, participating hospitals which have been accredited by the Joint Commission on Accreditation of Hospitals. The Secretary may in addition prescribe higher standards than required by accreditation by the Commission.

Conformation of Skilled Care Services and Facilities Under Medicare and Medicaid.   Skilled care services are similarly defined with respect to both Medicare and Medicaid, and standards of skilled nursing facilities are to be the same under both programs. The term *extended care facility* is eliminated.[53]

Professional Standards Review. This is the most extensive and important of the provisions directed to the problems of cost and quality control and medical necessity of services.[54] A new part (B) *Professional Standards Review* is added to Title XI of the Social Security Act. Provision is made for the establishment of *Professional Standards Review Organizations* within states for the review of the professional activities of physicians and other practitioners, and institutional and other providers of services in designated geographical areas.[55] These organizations are to be associations of physicians and open to and representative of physicians in the area. (After January 1, 1976, and then only if there is no such organization meeting the specified conditions, other competent agencies or organizations may be designated.)

Statewide Professional Standards Review Councils and a National Professional Standards Review Council are also to be established.

Social Services in Skilled Nursing Facilities. It is no longer to be required under Medicare that medical social services be furnished in a skilled nursing facility.

Chiropractic Services. Chiropractors' services are covered under Medicare and Medicaid with respect to treatment by means of manual manipulation of the spine; in the case of Medicare, this is specifically to be for correction of a subluxation demonstrated by X-ray.

Speech Pathology Services. Speech pathology is covered as a part of outpatient physical therapy services under Medicare.

Termination of Medical Assistance Advisory Council. The Medical Assistance Advisory Council is terminated and its Title IX advisory functions added to those of the Health Insurance Benefits Advisory Council.

---

[53] Extended care facilities are now termed *skilled nursing facilities.*

[54] The declared purpose of this section is to assure "that the services for which payment may be made under the Social Security Act will conform to appropriate professional standards and that payment for such services will be made—(1) only when, and to the extent, medically necessary . . ." and (2) in the case of inpatient services, only when these cannot "effectively be provided on an outpatient basis or more economically in a health care facility of a different type."

[55] The review of services provided other than in institutions will be at the option of the organization and subject to the approval of the Secretary.

Review of Care in Intermediate Care Facilities. The requirements for professional review of care and placement of patients are extended to intermediate care facilities.

Psychiatric Hospital Care for Individuals Under 21. Inpatient psychiatric hospital services under Medicaid are extended, under specified conditions, to persons under age 21.

Public Information concerning Survey Reports. The pertinent findings of surveys of health care institutions and agencies with regard to compliance with conditions of participation under Medicare are to be made available to the public.

Family Planning Services. Family planning services are added to the basic services which must be made available under Medicaid.

Penalty for Failure to Provide Child Health Screening under Medicaid. The matching funds to the states under Medicaid will be reduced by 1 percent where the states do not implement the previous requirements for providing for child health screening and subsequent corrective treatment services for children in families receiving aid to dependent children.[56]

Home Health Services Coinsurance. Coinsurance payments for home health services under Part B are eliminated.

Treatment for Chronic Renal Disease. Persons insured under Social Security, and their dependents, who require hemodialysis or renal transplantation for chronic renal disease are deemed disabled for purpose of coverage under Title XVIII, beginning 3 months after initiation of a course of renal dialysis. Reimbursement is to be limited to treatment centers meeting specified requirements.

Title III. Supplemental Security Income For the Aged, Blind and Disabled

This title creates, effective January 1, 1974, a new federal minimum income program (under a new Title XVI) to replace the federally aided adult public assistance programs. Grants to the states for social services for these groups will be continued under a new Title VI. (No change is made in the federal-state programs of aid to families with dependent children.)

---

[56] The programs established under these provisions have come to be known as Early and Periodic Screening, Diagnosis and Treatment (EPSDT) programs.

Title IV. Miscellaneous

This title includes provision for increased grants to the states for child welfare services.

10. SUMMARY OF MEDICARE

Title XVIII. Health Insurance for the Aged and Disabled

Part A. Hospital Insurance

Benefits

Hospital Inpatient Services

- Up to 90 days during any spell of illness.[57] Deductible ($92) and coinsurance ($23 per day after the sixtieth hospital day).[58]
- Lifetime reserve—60 days. ($46 coinsurance).[58]
- Lifetime limit for inpatient psychiatric care—90 days.

Post-Hospital Extended Care Services[59]

- Up to 100 days during any spell of illness. Coinsurance ($11.50 per day[58] after the twentieth day.)
- Three-day prior hospital admission required
- Continuing *skilled nursing care* or other skilled rehabilitation services must be needed for a condition for which the preceding inpatient services were received.

Post-Hospital Home Health Services

- Up to 100 visits in a one-year period, and related services and supplies.
- Skilled nursing care or physical or speech therapy must be needed for a condition for which the inpatient services were received. Services to be rendered under a plan established and periodically reviewed by a physician.

[57] Also referred to as a "benefit period".

[58] Deductible and coinsurance figures as of April 1976

[59] In a skilled nursing facility.

Exclusions

Private duty nurses
Cost of first three pints of blood

Financing

A special earnings tax on employees, employers and self-employed persons.

Conditions of Participation

Include utilization review plans for hospitals and skilled nursing facilities.

Part B. Supplementary Medical Insurance

Benefits

Physicians' Services

- Services of doctors of medicine and osteopathy, including professional services of hospital-based specialists (radiologists and pathologists)
- Limited, specified services by dentists, podiatrists, optometrists and chiropractors

Hospital Outpatient Services

Diagnostic Procedures

- Laboratory and X-ray services

Home Health Services

- Up to 100 visits in a one-year period. Conditions essentially the same as for Part A services, except for prior hospitalization.

Outpatient Physical Therapy and Speech Pathology Services

- Services rendered under the direct supervision of a physician or under certain circumstances as a part of home health services

Other Medical and Health Services

- Supplies, equipment, prostheses, radiation therapy, ambulance services (only, and under limited conditions, to a hospital or skilled nursing facility)

Deductibles and Coinsurance

Deductible is $60 per year; coinsurance is 20 percent of charges. (No deductible or coinsurance for home health services or radiologists' and pathologists' services to inpatients.)

Exclusions

Glasses, dentures, hearing aids, drugs, check-ups, dental care, routine foot care.

$250 annual limit on out of hospital psychiatric services

Financing

Monthly premium ($6.30) plus government matching

Administration

Social Security Administration: Bureau of Health, Insurance Public Health Service (certain specific functions, including standards)

Advisory Council

Health Insurance Benefits Advisory Council

II. SUMMARY OF MEDICAID

Title XIX. Grants to States for Medical Assistance Programs

Federal matching grants are made available, at the option of the states, for a single medical assistance program for:

- Recipients of federally aided public assistance[60]
- Recipients of supplemental security income benefits
- Medically indigent in comparable groups (families with dependent children, as defined for purposes of public assistance, and the aged, blind and disabled)

---

[60] Prior to January 1, 1974, the federally aided public assistance groups were families with dependent children (children deprived of parental support due to death, absence or incapacity of a parent, or, in certain circumstances, unemployment of the father), and indigent aged, blind, and disabled. The latter three groups are now under the federal supplemental security income program.

- Other needy children

States participating in the Medicaid program must include both the first and second categories above.

Programs are to include (some of each of) five basic services[61]

- Inhospital services
- Outpatient hospital services
- Other laboratory and X-ray services
- Skilled nursing home services
- Physicians' services

Also to be included by each participating state are:

- A program for screening of children for defects and chronic conditions, and appropriate treatment
- Family planning services

The states may also optionally include virtually any additional medical care services.

Federal matching: 50–83 percent of costs (according to state's per capita income)

All states have established Medicaid programs.

Administration

Social and Rehabilitation Service (Medical Assistance Administration)

State Agency—usually the department of public welfare

Advisory Council

Health Insurance Benefits Advisory Council

12. SUMMARY OF THE SOCIAL SECURITY ACT TITLES

Title I   *Grants to States for Old Age Assistance and Medical Assistance for the Aged**

Repealed

---

[61] Alternatively, (for medically indigent) states could select seven among these and other services (See appendix E). States including skilled nursing home services must also include home health services.

*Prior to January 1, 1974, there were four federally aided public assistance

| *Title II* | *Federal Old Age, Survivors and Disability Insurance Benefits* |

Title III — *Grants to States for Unemployment Compensation Administration*

Title IV — *Grants to States for Aid and Services to Needy Families with Children and for Child Welfare Services*

Title V — *Maternal and Child Health and Crippled Children's Services*

Title VI — *Grants to States for Services to the Aged, Blind or Disabled**

Repealed

Title VII — *Administration*

Provides for the administration of the Act by the Secretary of HEW and the Commissioner of Social Security. This Title also authorizes training grants for public welfare personnel.

Title VIII — *Taxes with Respect to Employment*

These provisions are now in the Internal Revenue Code

Title IX — *Miscellaneous Provisions Relating to Employment Security*

Title X — *Grants to States for Aid to the Blind**

Repealed

Title XI — *General Provisions and Professional Standards Review*

Title XII — *Advances to States' Unemployment Funds*

Title XIII — *Reconversion Unemployment Benefits for Seamen*

Expired

("welfare") categories. These were: Old Age Assistance (OAA), Aid to Families with Dependent Children (AFDC), Aid to the Blind (AB), and Aid to the Permanently and Totally Disabled (APTD).

Under provisions of the 1972 Social Security Amendments the three adult assistance categories (OAA, AB, APTD) became part of a new federal income supplement program (Supplemental Security Income, SSI) under a new Title VI. Titles I, X and XIV were repealed, (except with respect to Puerto Rico, Guam and the Virgin Islands).

Grants to the states for social services for the aged, blind and disabled were continued under a new Title VI. (The original provisions of Title VI, Public Health Work, had been transferred to the Public Health Services Act in 1944.) With the addition of Title XX, Grants to States for Services, Title VI was repealed.

Title XIV   Grants to States for Aid to the Permanently and Totally Disabled*

Repealed

Title XV   Unemployment Compensation for Federal Employees and the Ex-Servicemen's Unemployment Compensation Program

Repealed. These provisions are codified elsewhere.

Title XVI   Supplemental Security Income for the Aged, Blind and Disabled*

Title XVII   Grants for Planning Comprehensive Action to Combat Mental Retardation

Expired

Title XVIII   Health Insurance for the Aged and Disabled

"Medicare"

Title XIX   Grants to States for Medical Assistance Programs

"Medicaid"

Title XX   Grants to States for Services*

Administration

OASDI program—*Social Security Administration*
Public Assistance and Medical Assistance (Medicaid)—*Social and Rehabilitation Service*
Medicare—*Social Security Administration* and *Public Health Service*
Maternal and Child Health—*Public Health Service* (*Health Services Administration*)
Unemployment Insurance—*Department of Labor*
Supplemental Security Income—*Social Security Administration*

13. THE PUBLIC HEALTH SERVICE ACT

An Act to consolidate and revise the laws relating to the Public Health Service and for other purposes.

The Public Health Service Act of 1944 revised and brought together in one statute all existing legislation concerning the Public Health Service (including Title VI of the Social Security Act). It set forth provisions for the organization, staffing, and activities of the Service.

It has subsequently been the vehicle, by amendment, of a number of important federal grant-in-aid programs.

Title I. Short Title and Definitions

Titles I through V may be cited as the "Public Health Service Act."

Title II. Administration

General organization of the Public Health Service. It shall be administered by the Surgeon General under the direction of the Federal Security Administrator. The Service shall consist of: (1) the Office of the Surgeon General, (2) the National Institute of Health, (3) the Bureau of Medical Services, and (4) the Bureau of State Services.

Grades, ranks, and titles of the Commissioned Corps, and relevant policies and regulations.[62]

Organization and duties of the National Advisory Health Council and National Advisory Cancer Council.

Title III. General Powers and Duties of the Public Health Service

Part A. Research and Investigations

Sec. 301   The Service shall conduct, encourage, cooperate in, and promote research and investigations relating to physical and mental diseases and impairments.

Sec. 302   In carrying out the purposes of this section with regard to narcotics, activities shall include studies and investigations regarding the use and misuse of narcotic drugs. The Surgeon General shall give aid and advice to state officials in the care, treatment, and rehabilitation of narcotics addicts.

Part B. Federal-State Cooperation

Sec. 311   The Surgeon General is authorized to accept from and provide *assistance to state and local authorities* in prevention and control of communicable diseases.

---

[62] Commissioned officers include personnel in "medicine, surgery, dentistry, hygiene, sanitary engineering, pharmacy, nursing, or related scientific specialties in public health."

Sec. 312   A *health conference* of the state health authorities shall be called annually.[63]

Sec. 313   Collection and compilation of *vital statistics.*

Sec. 314   Grants and services to the states to assist in *venereal disease control, tuberculosis control,* and the establishment and maintenance of adequate *state and local public health services.*

Annual allotments to the states shall be made on the basis of: (1) population, (2) the size of the venereal dissease and tuberculosis problems and other special health problems and (3) the financial need of the respective states.

Grants shall be paid on the condition that the states spend for the same general purpose from its funds an amount determined in accordance with regulations.

Regulations and amendments regarding grants to the states shall be made after consultation with a conference of the state health authorities; the Surgeon General shall obtain insofar as practicable the agreement of the state health authorities prior to the issuance of such regulations or amendments.

Sec. 315   The Surgeon General shall issue from time to time *information related to public health,* including publications for the public, weekly reports on health conditions, and other pertinent information for those engaged in work related to the functions of the Service.

Part C. Hospitals, Medical Examinations, and Medical Care

Sec. 322   Management and operation of the institutions, hospitals, and stations of the Service. Medical care to be provided for *merchant seamen* and certain other persons.[64]

Sec. 323   The Service is to furnish medical services in *penal and correctional* institutions of the United States.

Sec. 324   The Surgeon General is authorized to provide medical

[63] Known as the Conference of State and Territorial Health Officers.

[64] Including members of the U.S. Maritime Service, Merchant Marine cadets, quarantine and immigration detainees.

services to *federal employees* and longshoremen for work-related illness or injury and medical examinations for employees and retirees.

Sec. 325   Medical examination of *aliens.*

Sec. 326   Members of the Coast Guard, Coast and Geodetic Survey and the Commissioned Corps of the Public Health Service are entitled to *treatment and hospitalization by the Service.*

Part D. Lepers

Sec. 331–   The Public Health Service shall receive and care for per-
332   sons with leprosy.

Part E. Narcotics Addicts

Sec. 341–   Care and treatment, in hospitals of the Service, of narcot-
345   ics addicts who are federal prisoners or who voluntarily request treatment.

Part F. Biological Products

Sec. 351–   Regulation of the manufacture, labeling, and sale of
352   biological products (virus, serum, toxin, anti-toxin, or other product) applicable to the prevention or cure of disease or injuries of man.

Part G. Quarantine and Inspection

Sec. 361–   Inspection, quarantine, and other procedures necessary
367   to prevent transmission or spread of communicable diseases from foreign countries into states or possessions or from one state or possession into another.

Title IV. National Cancer Institute[65]

The National Cancer Institute shall be a division of the National Institute of Health, to carry out the purposes of Part A or Title III (Research and Investigation) with regard to cancer. It is to:

1. Conduct and assist researches, investigations and studies relating to the cause, prevention and treatment of cancer.

[65] This title in effect re-enacted the National Cancer Act of 1937.

2. Promote the coordination of researches conducted by the Institute and similar researches conducted by other agencies and individuals.
3. Provide training and instruction in technical matters relating to diagnoses and treatment of cancer.
4. Provide fellowships in the Institute.
5. Secure for the Institute consultation service and advice of cancer experts from the United States and abroad.
6. Cooperate with state health agencies in prevention, control and eradication of cancer.
7. Procure, use, and lend radium for purposes of this Title.

Grants-in-aid for cancer projects shall be made only after review and recommendations of the National Cancer Advisory Council.

This Title is not to be construed as limiting the functions or authority of the Surgeon General or the Public Health Service under any other Title of this Act relating to the study of the prevention, diagnosis and treatment of cancer.

Title V. Miscellaneous

Miscellaneous regulations, and authorization for the *admission to St. Elizabeths Hospital* of insane patients entitled to treatment by the Service.

Amendments to the Public Health Service Act

There have been many amendments to the Public Health Service Act. Several are of particular interest:

The Hospital Survey and Construction Act of 1946 (Hill-Burton Act) inaugurated the Hill-Burton program of health facilities construction.

The Health Amendments of 1956 (grants for training in public health and nursing) initiated the program of federal assistance for education and training of health personnel which has been gradually extended and broadened by subsequent legislation to many categories of health personnel and institutions. A recent and important example is the *Comprehensive Health Manpower Act of 1971*.

The Heart Disease, Cancer and Stroke Amendments of 1965—established the Regional Medical Programs.

The Comprehensive Health Planning Amendments of 1966 ("Partnership for Health")— designed to give the states more flexibility in use of their grants-in-aid for public health work and to encourage comprehensive health planning; it was the base for the state and area-wide comprehensive health planning "A" and "B" agencies.

The Health Maintenance Organization Act of 1973—established a program of financial assistance for the development of health maintenance organizations.

National Health Planning and Resources Development Act of 1974— consolidated and greatly revised the Hill-Burton, regional medical programs and comprehensive health planning legislation.

These amendments are described more fully in subsequent sections.

Other noteworthy amending Acts are:

Health Services for Agricultural Migratory Workers (1962). This Act established a program of grants for family clinics and other health services for migrant workers.

Communicable Disease Control Amendments of 1970. This legislation re-established the categorical grant program for control of communicable diseases, including tuberculosis, venereal disease, rubella, measles, Rh disease, poliomyelitis, diphtheria, tetanus and whooping cough.

Family Planning Services and Population Research Act of 1970. This established an Office of Population Affairs under the Assistant Secretary for Health and Scientific Affairs. It added Title X, *Population Research and Voluntary Family Planning Programs*, to the Public Health Service Act. This authorized project, formula and training grants and contracts for family planning programs and services (abortion excepted), and research grants and contracts in fields related to family planning and population.

Emergency Health Personnel Act of 1970. This Act authorized the Secretary to assign commissioned officers and other health personnel of the Public Health Service to areas designated as in critical need of health manpower. It provided a statutory base for the National Health Service Corps.

National Sickle Cell Anemia Control Act (1972). This added a new Title XI to the Public Health Service Act: *Sickle Cell Anemia Program.* It authorized grants and contracts for screening and counseling, research, and informational programs related to sickle cell anemia.

National Cooley's Anemia Control Act (1972). Title XI was changed to *Genetic Blood Disorders* and Part B, *Cooley's Anemia Programs*, was added. This authorized grants and contracts for Cooley's anemia screening, treatment and counseling, research, and educational programs.

Communicable Disease Control Amendments of 1972. This Act extended the programs of grants for communicable disease control and established a separate one for prevention and control of venereal disease.

Health Programs Extension Act of 1973. This Act extended through June 30, 1974 a number of programs whose authorizations were due to expire. These included migrant health, comprehensive health planning, Hill-Burton, allied health manpower training, regional medical programs and family planning programs as well as programs under the Community Mental Health Centers Act and the Developmental Disabilities Services and Facilities Construction Act.

Emergency Medical Services Systems Act of 1973. This added a new title to the Public Health Service Act: Title XII—*Emergency Medical Services Systems.* It established a program of grants and contracts for the development and improvement of area emergency medical services systems, and for related research and training.

Sudden Infant Death Syndome Act of 1974. Part C, *Sudden Infant Death Syndrome* was added to Title XI; this provides for public and professional informational programs related to this syndrome.

Public Health Service Act Amendments (1975).[66] This omnibus Act extended and revised a number of health programs and activities: comprehensive public health services[67] (Special Health Revenue Sharing Act of 1975); family planning (Family Planning and Population Research Act of 1975); migrant health; community health centers; National Health Service Corps and nurse training (Nurse Training Act

[66] Passed over Presidential veto

[67] Services provided under Section 314d (See p. 175)

of 1975). Part D, *Hemophilia Programs* was added to Title XI, providing for projects for the development of diagnostic and treatment centers and blood component separation centers. (This Act also incorporated the Community Mental Health Centers Amendments of 1975.)

14. HOSPITAL SURVEY AND CONSTRUCTION ACT OF 1946* "HILL-BURTON ACT"

"An Act to amend the Public Health Service Act to authorize grants to the States for surveying their hospital and public health centers and for planning construction of additional facilities, and to authorize grants to assist in such construction."

This Act established the first of many post-World War II federally aided health programs.

Background

There was relatively little hospital construction during the years of the Great Depression and World War II. In 1944 a Commission on Hospital Care was organized by the American Hospital Association and the Public Health Service to study the national need for hospital facilities. The principles developed by the Commission and the Public Health Service are reflected in the Survey and Construction Act, introduced by Senators Hill and Burton, which became Title VI of the Public Health Service Act.

Summary of Major Provisions[68]

- Grants to assist the states to *inventory* their existing hospitals and health centers and to *survey* the need and develop programs for the construction of such facilities.
- Grants to the states for *construction projects.*
- Federal funds for surveys and planning to be allotted to the states on the *basis of population.* Within its allotment, a state may receive a grant equal to 33-1/3 percent of these expenses.

Funds for construction to be allotted annually to the states in

---

*PL 79-725

[68] The general language of this Act is representative of legislation authorizing grants-in-aid to the states.

accordance with a *formula* based on population and per capita income; from this allotment, grants may be made covering 33-1/3 percent of the cost of construction projects.

- In order to receive funds, a state must (among other provisions):
  a. Designate a *single state agency* to administer or supervise administration of the program, and establish a *state advisory council* to consult with the state agency. The council to include representatives of nongovernmental agencies and state agencies concerned with hospitals, and representatives of the *consumers* of hospital services.
  b. Submit a *state plan* for the construction of facilities based on the state-wide survey of need and conforming to regulations prescribed by the Surgeon General.
  c. Provide for the designation of a State Advisory Council to consult with the State Agency in carrying out the Act's purposes.
- The Surgeon General shall develop regulations concerning:
  a. The number of general hospital beds required to provide adequate hospital services in a state and the general methods by which such beds would be distributed. (Total beds for any state not to exceed 4.5 per thousand population, except up to 5.5 beds per thousand in less populated states.)
  b. The number of tuberculosis, mental disease, and chronic disease hospital beds required, and their distribution.
  c. The number and distribution of public health centers.
  d. The general manner in which the state agency will determine priorities for projects within a state, with special consideration to be given to hospital serving *rural communities.*
  e. General *standards* for construction and equipment for hospitals.
  f. Requirements that the State plan provide for adequate hospital facilities for State residents without discrimination and for persons unable to pay therefor.[69]
- Grants are to be available only to states who enact or have enacted legislation providing for minimum standards of maintenance and operation for hospitals receiving federal aid under this program.
- The Surgeon General is to consult with a *Federal Hospital Council* in administration of this title. The council shall consist of eight members (plus the Surgeon General), including four representatives of consumers of hospital services.

By 1949, all the states and territories had had state plans approved

---

[69] This section has been the subject of important litigation, with regard to racial segregation (see 1964 amendments) and the issue of provision of health care to the poor.

by the Surgeon General. In most instances, the state health department had been designated as the responsible agency for the administration of the program. Most states now had licensure laws, most of which were applicable to all hospitals, not just those eligible for federal aid.

Hill-Burton Amendments

The Hill-Burton Act has been amended frequently since its original enactment.

The *Hospital Survey and Construction Amendments of 1949* extended the program, increased the authorized funds and provided that the federal share of the costs of construction projects could be as much as 66-2/3 percent, depending on the relative need and economic status of the area involved. Additionally, grants were authorized for *research and demonstrations* relating to the development, utilization and coordination of hospital services and facilities.[70]

The *Medical Facilities Survey and Construction Act of 1954* authorized grants for surveys and for construction of *diagnostic and treatment* centers (including hospital OPDs), *chronic disease* hospitals, rehabilitation facilities and nursing homes.

Chronic disease hospitals were already included in the existing program, as were the other types of facilities when part of a hospital. The purpose of the legislation was to encourage the construction of such facilities by specifically earmarking funds for them and by including them though not part of a hospital.

The *Community Health Services and Facilities Act of 1961*, which dealt primarily with the question of improving out of hospital services for the aged and chronically ill, included several amendments to the Hill-Burton program. Funds for *nursing home* construction were increased and the hospital research and demonstration grant program was extended to other medical facilities.

The *Hospital and Medical Facilities Amendments of 1964* extended the program and authorized grants specifically earmarked for *modernization* of hospitals with more priority being given to urban areas.[71]

A new category of long-term care facilities was created which

---

[70] However, no funds were actually appropriated under this authorization until 1956.

combined the chronic disease hospitals and nursing home categories, and its funding authorization was increased.

A state was now permitted to use up to 2 percent of its allotment (up to $50,000) for half the *costs of administration* of the program.

Grants were authorized to the state agencies for up to 50 percent of the costs of comprehensive regional or local area *plans* for coordination of existing and planned health facilities. (Planning to be done by state agencies or by designated local public or nonprofit groups.)

Language was added requiring that "any facility or portion thereof to be constructed or modernized, [is] to be made available to all persons residing in the territorial area of the applicant." This replaced the previous "separate . . . if like quality" provisions.[72]

The *Medical Facilities Construction and Modernization Amendments of 1970*[73] again extended the program and added new provisions for federal loans and loan guarantees for construction and modernization. A new program of project grants was established for emergency rooms, communications networks, and transportation systems.

The *National Health Planning and Resources Development Act of 1974* revised the Hill-Burton legislation and incorporated it in a new Title XVI.

Administration

Health Resources Administration (Bureau of Health Planning and Resources Development)

15. HEART DISEASE, CANCER AND STROKE AMENDMENTS OF 1965* "REGIONAL MEDICAL PROGRAMS"

"An Act to amend the Public Health Service Act to assist in combatting heart disease, cancer, stroke, and related diseases."

[71] Authority for modernization existed in previous legislation but priority was given to "hospitals serving rural communities and areas with relatively small financial resources."

[72] A federal court had ruled (1963) this clause unconstitutional (Moses H. Cone Memorial Hospital *vs.* Simkins); the Supreme Court refused (1964) to review this decision, thus in effect barring racial segregation in hospitals receiving federal funds under the Hill-Burton program.

[73] Passed over Presidential veto.

*PL 89-239

This legislation reflects the general goals expressed in the 1964 report of the President's Commission on Heart Disease, Cancer and Stroke, although the recommendations were much modified.

Title IX is added to the Public Health Service Act. Its purposes are:

". . . to encourage and assist in the establishment of regional cooperative arrangements among medical schools, research institutions, and hospitals for research and training (including continuing education) and for related demonstrations of patient care in the fields of heart disease, cancer, stroke and related diseases:

"to afford the medical profession and the medical institutions of the nation, through such cooperative arrangements, the opportunity of making available to their patients the latest advances in the diagnosis and treatment of these diseases,

". . . and to accomplish these ends without interfering with the patterns, or the methods of financing, of patient care or professional practice or with the administration of hospitals. . . ."

Summary of Major Provisions

Grants are authorized to assist universities, medical schools, research institutions and other institutions and agencies in *planning* the development of regional medical programs and in *establishment and operation* of such programs.

A *regional medical program* is defined as a cooperative arrangement among a group of institutions or agencies engaged in research, training, diagnosis and treatment relating to heart disease, cancer or stroke, and, at the option of the applicant, related diseases. This group must:

- Be situated within an appropriate geographic area (which may be composed of part of parts of one or more states)
- Consist of one or more medical centers, one or more clinical research centers, and one or more hospitals[74]
- Have in effect adequate cooperative arrangements

---

[74] "A *medical center* means a medical school or other medical institution involved in postgraduate medical training and one or more affiliated hospitals."

A *clinical research center* means an institution (or part of an institution) the primary function of which is research and training of specialists and which, in connection therewith, provides specialized diagnostic and treatment services.

A *hospital* means "a health facility in which local capability for diagnosis and treatment is supported and augmented by the program established under this title."

An applicant must designate an *advisory group* to advise the applicant (and the participating institutions and agencies) regarding the planning and operation of the regional medical program. The advisory group is to include practicing physicians, medical center officials, hospital administrators, and representatives from appropriate organizations and institutions.

- A *National Advisory Council on Regional Medical Programs* is established.

Regional Medical Programs Amendments

The *Public Health Service Amendments of 1968* extended the regional medical programs and made several adjustments and clarifications.

Extensive additions and changes were made in the *Public Health Service Amendments of 1970*. These extended the program for three years and (among other provisions):

- Broadened the scope of the program by adding *kidney disease* as one of the diseases to which the program is specifically addressed; Title IX now to read ". . . Stroke, Kidney Disease and Other Related Diseases."
- Further broadened and clarified the purposes of the Title:
  a. To explicitly include *medical data exchange* among the activities of the programs
  b. To make explicit that *prevention* and *rehabilitation* as well as diagnosis and treatment are program concerns
  c. "To promote and foster linkages among health care institutions and providers so as to strengthen and improve *primary care* and the relationship between specialized and primary care"
  d. "To improve health services for persons residing in areas with limited health services"
- Required official health and *health planning* agency representation on the *advisory groups* and that public members include persons familiar with the financing of, as well as the need for, services and that such public members be sufficient in numbers to insure adequate community orientation of regional medical programs.
- Required that the appropriate regional metropolitan or local *areawide comprehensive health planning agency* (authorized under Section 314b) have an opportunity to consider (for example, review and comment on) any operational grant proposal or applica-

tion of a regional medical program involving facilities, services or functions within that areawide agency's jurisdiction.

- Authorized *training grants* for training health manpower in the areas included in the legislation, and permitted support of research, studies, investigations and demonstrations designed to maximize the utilization of manpower in the deliver of health services.
- Specifically permitted funds to be used for special projects for improving and developing new means for the *delivery of health services* concerned with heart disease, cancer, stroke, kidney disease, and other related diseases.

By 1971 there were 56 regional medical programs covering all the states and trust territories. Most encompassed single states but some incorporated two or more states, parts of two or more states, or parts of single states.[75]

With the passage of the *National Health Planning and Resources Development Act of 1974*, the regional medical programs as such are no longer funded as separate entities.

16. COMPREHENSIVE HEALTH PLANNING AND PUBLIC HEALTH SERVICE AMENDMENTS OF 1966* "PARTNERSHIP FOR HEALTH"

"An Act to amend the Public Health Service Act to promote and assist in the extension and improvement of comprehensive health planning and public health services, [and] to provide for a more effective use of available Federal funds for such planning and services . . ."

Background

In the years since the passage of the Public Health Service Act of 1944 the program of grants to the states for public health work had been expended largely by designating funds for specific purposes. As of 1966, most of the federal support to the states for public health services was made available through one or another of such "categorical

[75] For example, Tri-State Regional Medical Program (Massachusetts, New Hampshire, and Rhode Island), Intermountain Regional Medical Program (Utah and parts of Colorado, Idaho, Montana, Nevada, and Wyoming), and Western New York Regional Medical Program.

*PL 89-749

grants."[76] This system had come under considerable criticism, as being excessively rigid, denying the state health department freedom to determine the allocation of these funds to public health problems. This legislation represents a departure from this approach to funding of public health services; it authorizes "block" grants for public health programs and includes provisions for the development of state and local planning for comprehensive health services.

These amendments essentially involved a complete revision of Section 314 (Title III) which now referred to grants for *Comprehensive Health Planning* and for *Comprehensive Public Health Services*.

Summary of Major Provisions

Sec. 314a *Grants to the States for Comprehensive State Health Planning*

In order to qualify for these funds, a state is to submit a "plan for comprehensive state health planning." This plan must designate a state agency (new or existing) to be responsible for the state's health planning functions, and provide for the establishment of a *state health planning* council to advise this agency. The council is to include representatives of state and local agencies, nongovernmental organizations and groups, and consumers of health services; a majority of the membership are to be representatives of consumers.

The plan further is to provide for "encouraging cooperative efforts among governmental or nongovernmental agencies, organizations and groups concerned with health services, facilities, or manpower," and for cooperative efforts between them and similar agencies, organizations, and groups in the fields of education, welfare, and rehabilitation.

Sec. 314b *Project Grants for Areawide Health Planning*

Grants are authorized, with the consent of the above state agency, to any other public or nonprofit agency or organization "for developing comprehensive regional, metropolitan area or other local area plans for coordination of existing and planned health services, including facilities and persons required for provision of such services."[77]

---

[76] Among these were cancer, chronic illness, dental disease, heart disease, mental illness, tuberculosis, and venereal disease.

[77] The state planning agency became known as the "A" agency; the sub-state agency, the "B" or "areawide" agency (or, "314a" and "314b" agencies).

Federal share: 75 percent of the costs of such projects.

Sec. 314c *Project Grants for Training, Studies, and Demonstrations*

Grants to agencies, institutions, or other organizations for projects for training, studies and demonstrations relating to the development of improved or more effective comprehensive health planning.

Sec. 314d *Grants for Comprehensive Public Health Services*

Grants to "assist the states in establishing and maintaining adequate public health services, including the training of personnel for state and local health work." Again to qualify for these funds, state plans for the provision of public health services are required and these plans are to be developed in accordance with the plan for comprehensive health planning. The federal share for public health programs under this section is to be 33-1/3 to 66-2/3 percent, and at least 15 percent of a state's allotment is to be used for mental health services.

Sec. 314e *Project Grants for Health Services Development*[78]

Grants are authorized to public or nonprofit private agencies, institutions or organizations to cover part of the cost of

- Providing services to meet health needs of limited geographic scope or of specialized regional or national significance;
- Stimulating and supporting, for an initial period, new programs of health services;
- Undertaking studies, demonstrations or training designed to develop new methods or improve existing methods of providing health services

Comprehensive Health Planning Amendments

The *Partnership for Health Amendments of 1967* extended the program and made several additions and modifications including:

- State plans for comprehensive health planning are to provide for assisting each state health institution to develop a program for capital expenditures for replacement, modernization and expansion consistent with meeting the needs of the state for facilities and services most economically, efficiently, and without duplication.
- Representation of the *interests of local government* in areawide planning agencies is required.

[78] The intent of this section, also, was to provide more flexibility in the use of such project grants than had formerly been the case.

- After July 1, 1968, 70 percent of the states' grant funds must be available for *services in communities* of the states (i.e., locally).

The *Public Health Service Amendments of 1970* extended the program for an additional three years and made several further modifications:

- State and areawide plans must include *home health services.*
- The state planning agency could receive a grant under Section 314b if no application for a grant for the region involved has been filed by any other qualified organization.
- Areawide health planning councils are to be established to include representatives of the interests of local government, of the regional medical programs and of *consumers* of health services. A majority of the members of such councils are to be representatives of consumers.

The *National Health Planning and Resources Development Act of 1974* completely revised the comprehensive health planning program as Title XV—National Health Planning and Development.

17. HEALTH MANPOWER LEGISLATION UNDER THE PUBLIC HEALTH SERVICE ACT

The first federal legislation particularly addressed to the question of health manpower, except for certain temporary wartime programs, was the *Health Amendments Act of 1956.* This law authorized under Title III of the Public Health Service Act traineeship for professional public health personnel[79] and for advanced training of professional nurses. A third provision amended the Vocational Education Act of 1946 to authorize grants for programs for practical nurse training.[80]

A program of formula grants to *schools of public health* was established in 1958. (PL 85-544).[81] In 1960 there was added (PL 86-720) a program of project grants to schools of public health and schools of nursing or engineering providing graduate or specialized public health training. The *Graduate Public Health Training Amendments of 1964*

---

[79] Physicians, engineers, nurses and other professional health personnel.

[80] Such training had been permitted under the general vocational education program, but this amendment made specific provisions for this.

[81] By earmarking for this purpose a portion of the funds authorized to the states for public health services. In 1966 (PL 89-749) the program was separately provided for.

broadened eligibility for project grants to include other institutions providing such training.

Health Professions Education Assistance Act of 1963

This Act inaugurated, under Title VII of the Public Health Service Act, the program of *construction grants* for teaching facilities: grants for the construction or rehabilitation of facilities for training of physicians, dentists, pharmacists, podiatrists, nurses,[82] or professional public health personnel, these contigent on increased first year enrollments. Also authorized was a program of *student loan funds* at schools of medicine, osteopathy, and dentistry.[83]

Nurse Training Act of 1964

This Act added Title VIII, "Nurse Training," to the Public Health Service Act. This authorized separate funding for construction grants for schools of nursing and extended eligibility to associate degree and diploma schools; these were also contingent on increased enrollment. Also authorized were project grants to the schools to improve and expand their training programs, and formula grants to diploma schools.[84] Provision was also made for the establishment of *student loan funds* at schools of nursing.

Health Professions Assistance Amendments of 1965

These amendments authorized a program of grants to "improve the quality of schools of medicine, dentistry, osteopathy, optometry and podiatry." These were *basic improvement* (institutional) grants related to enrollment and contingent on increased enrollment, and *special improvement* grants. *Scholarship* grants were also authorized for these schools, plus schools of pharmacy. The student loan program was expanded, with provisions for partial cancellation for

[82] In schools with baccalaureate or graduate degree programs.

[83] Following the general pattern of loan funds established under the National Defense Education Act of 1958. Students of optometry and veterinary medicine were subsequently included (PL 88-654, 89-709).

[84] Formula grants related to the number of "federally sponsored" students (those receiving loans from the fund also established), and to increased enrollment.

physicians, dentists, and optometrists practicing in shortage areas, and eligibility was extended to students of pharmacy and podiatry.

Allied Health Professions Personnel Training Act of 1966

This Act established programs of *construction* and *improvement grants* for training centers for allied health professions,[85] generally patterned after those in the previous legislation. For the construction grants, the facilitation of training in *three or more related* (of specified) curriculums was to be taken into account. *Advanced traineeships* for allied health professions personnel were authorized, as were project grants related to the training of new types of health technologists. Additional loan cancellation was provided for physicians, dentists, and optometrists practicing in poor rural areas. Revolving funds for loans to student loan funds were authorized under Titles VII and VIII and the latter title was further amended to authorize "opportunity grants for nursing education" (*scholarships* for nursing students of exceptional financial need), and contracts with agencies and institutions to identify such individuals and to publicize sources of financial aid.

Health Manpower Act of 1968

This Act extended, with some changes, most of the previous programs. Among the changes were the extension of the institutional and special project grants to schools of pharmacy and veterinary medicine and the addition of students of veterinary medicine to the scholarship program.[86] Also, the Secretary was directed to prepare a report on Title VII programs.

Health Training Improvement Act of 1970

This Act provided for institutional grants for new schools of health professions and directed the Secretary to report to Congress on the need for emergency financial assistance to medical and dental schools.

---

[85] Defined as a "junior college, college, or university which provides education leading to a baccalaureate or associate degree (or equivalents) or a higher degree in medical technology, dental hygiene, or other curriculums specified by regulations. . . ."

[86] These schools had become eligible for construction grants in 1966 (PL 89-709).

It extended, with some changes, the grant programs for allied health professions. Changes included broadening of eligibility for advanced traineeships to other organizations and institutions in addition to those defined as training centers. Authorization was added for *special project* grants and contracts related to training or retraining of allied health personnel. Also authorized was a program of grants and contracts for projects related to encouraging and assisting the entry into allied health professions training of individuals of financial, educational, or cultural need, and provision was made for grants for *scholarships, work-study programs*, and *student loan funds*. The Secretary was directed to conduct a study of the provisions and programs relating to allied health professions in the Public Health Service Act and other Acts, and also to report on the major problems associated with licensure, certification, and other qualifications for health personnel.

Comprehensive Health Manpower Training Act of 1971[87]

This Act extended the program of construction grants for health research and teaching facilities, raised the latter grant ceiling to 70–80 percent, and mandated an opportunity for review and comment by the appropriate 314a and 314b agencies. Provisions for construction loan guarantees and interest subsidies were added.

The previous institutional grants were replaced by a new system of *capitation grants* for each student enrolled in health professional schools, again contingent upon increased first-year enrollment and upon submission of plans for projects for improvement of teaching programs in at least three of nine specified categories.[88] *Start up*

---

[87] This is a particularly complex and important piece of legislation. Those with particular interest in the subject would be well advised to read the complete law and the House Committee report.

An extensive description and commentary on this and other recent health manpower legislation is found in *Federal Laws: Health/Environment Manpower*, by John T. Grupenhoff and Stephen P. Strickland (Washington, D.C.: Science and Communication Group, 1972).

[88] These covered such activities as curriculum improvements (including shortening), interdisciplinary training, training for new roles or types of personnel (including physician assistants and nurse practitioners), teaching of health care organization; training in clinical pharmacology, nutrition, and management of drug and alcohol abuse, programs related to admission and retention of disadvantaged students, and projects related to training primary care health professionals and family medicine.

assistance to new schools of medicine, osteopathy, and dentistry was authorized, also in the form of capitation grants.

Special project grants to health professions schools were authorized for a wide variety of activities related to professional education in priority areas and the utilization of health personnel; *contracts* were authorized with other health and educational entities for similar projects. Additionally, grants were authorized to schools in *financial distress*.

A new program of grants and contracts, *health manpower education initiative awards*, was authorized for health and educational entities to support a wide variety of projects for the purpose of "improving the distribution, supply, quality, utilization, and efficiency of health personnel and the health services delivery system;" these awards are to be coordinated with the area's regional medical program. Additional grants were authorized for special projects related to enrollment of students who might be expected to practice in shortage areas, and students who are financially or otherwise disadvantaged.

The *loan* provisions were broadened to provide up to 85 percent cancellation for health professionals practicing for three years in shortage areas. *Scholarships* for needy students were increased and provision was made for the total amounts available for the scholarship funds to be increased according to numbers of students enrolled from low income backgrounds. A new *physician shortage area* scholarship program was established for medical students who agree to practice primary care (one year for each scholarship year) in an area of physician shortage or with substantial numbers of migratory agricultural workers.

Another new program included grants for training, traineeships, and fellowships in family medicine; annual capitation grants for approved graduate training programs for physicians and dentists in primary care and other designated shortage areas of care; grants for advanced training, traineeships and fellowships for health professions teaching personnel; and grants related to the use of computer technology in health care.

Finally, there were a number of miscellaneous provisions relating to health manpower. A National Health Manpower Clearinghouse was established. The Secretary was directed to "use his best efforts to provide, to each county certified by him to be without the services of a physician . . . at least one physician in the Public Health

Service. . . .[89] The Comptroller General was directed to conduct a study of *health facilities construction costs.* The Secretary was directed to arrange for a study (preferably by the National Academy of Sciences) of the annual per student *educational cost* of schools of health professions (including nursing) and to prepare a report on the parts of Title VII related to health professionals education.

Nurse Training Act of 1971[90]

This Act extended the construction grant program, increased the grant ceiling to 67-75 percent, and added provisions for loan construction guarantees and interest subsidies. The program of special project grants was broadened to cover a wide variety of activities related to nursing and interdisciplinary training; contract authorization was added, and provision was made for grants to schools in *financial distress.*

The program of formula grants to diploma schools[91] was replaced by annual *capitation* grants for nursing schools, contingent on increased enrollment,[92] with additional amounts authorized for further enrollment increase, and for schools with training programs for nurse midwives, family health nurses, and other nurse practitioners. An additional requirement for these grants was that a school submit a plan to carry out projects in at least three of several categories related to improved nursing training, and the Secretary was directed to report to the appropriate Congressional committees on the carrying out of these projects. A separate program of *start up* grants was authorized for new nurse training programs.

The advanced traineeships and the student loan program were continued, with provision made for loan cancellation up to 85 percent after five years of full-time nursing employment, and, for practice in an area of shortage, up to 85 percent after three years. *Half-time* students were also made eligible for loans. The *scholarship* program was extended and expanded, with half-time students becoming eligible.

Additionally, grants and contracts were authorized to health or

[89] Amending the Emergency Personnel Act (National Health Service Corps).

[90] This is the companion to the Comprehensive Health Manpower Act and contains many analogous provisions.

[91] This program was not actually funded and thus was never implemented.

[92] Which could be waived if circumstances warranted.

educational entities for activities related to the enrollment in schools of nursing of persons such as veterans with health field experience, the financially and otherwise disadvantaged, and licensed practical nurses. Finally, the Secretary was directed to report to Congress on the administration and impact of the Title VIII programs.

Nurse Training Act of 1975[93]

This Act extended and revised the various programs related to nursing education and in addition made new grant and contract authorization for special projects including advanced nursing training and nurse practitioner programs, and cooperative arrangements (including mergers) among hospital training programs and academic institutions.

Administration

Health Resources Administration (Bureau of Health Manpower)

Advisory Councils

National Advisory Council on Health Professions Education
National Advisory Council on Nurse Training

Note

A large number of grant programs are authorized in this legislation. It should be kept in mind that the actual receipt of grants is dependent upon the level of funds actually appropriated by Congress, and the allocation of funds by the administrative agencies. As of this writing, passage of extensive new health manpower legislation is anticipated.

18. HEALTH MAINTENANCE ORGANIZATION ACT OF 1973*

"An Act to amend the Public Health Service Act to provide assistance and encouragement for the establishment and expansion of health maintenance organizations, and for other purposes."

A new title, XIII, *Health Maintenance Organizations*, is added to the Public Health Service Act.

[93] Title IX of PL 94-63
*PL 93-222

Summary of Major Provisions

Financial Assistance for the Development of Health Maintenance Organizations

There is established a program of financial assistance for the development or expansion of health maintenance organizations. This comprises:

- Grants and contracts to determine the feasibility of development or expansion of individual health maintenance organizations;
- Grants and contracts for planning projects;
- Grants, contracts and loan guarantees for initial development;
- Loans and loan guarantees for initial operating costs (to offset, when necessary, losses during the first 36 months.)

For purposes of this title, a health maintenance organization is a legal entity which provides basic and supplemental services to its members, and is organized and operated in a prescribed manner.

Basic medical services are to be provided for a set, periodic payment fixed under a community rating system. These services are:

- Physician services
- Inpatient and outpatient services
- Medically necessary emergency health services
- Short-term outpatient evaluative and crisis intervention mental health services (not over 20 visits)
- Medical treatment and referral services for alcohol and drug abuse
- Laboratory and X-ray services
- Home health services
- Preventive services (including voluntary family planning and infertility services, and preventive dental care and eye examination for children)

Nominal additional payments may be required for specific basic services.

The basic health services payment may be supplemented by nominal charges for specific services (copayment) unless this is determined to be an undue barrier to the delivery of health services.

Supplemental health services are to be made available to enrolled members who wish to contract for them. These are:

- Intermediate and long-term care
- Vision care and dental and mental health services not included under basic services

- Provision of prescription drugs

At least 20 percent of the appropriated funds are to be allocated to rural health maintenance organizations.

Professional services which are provided as basic services are in general to be provided through health professionals who are members of the staff of the health maintenance organizations or through medical groups or individual practice associations.

The requirements for a health maintenance organization include

- Evidence of fiscal responsibility
- Enrollment of persons broadly representative of the age, social and income groups within the area served; except that not more than 75 percent of the members may be enrolled from a medically underserved population, unless the area served is a rural area
- A policy making board, at least one-third of whose membership are (enrolled) members of the organization, and with equitable representation of the medically underserved population
- Arrangements for a quality assurance program
- Provision of medical social services and health education services
- Provision for continuing education for its health professional staff

Organizations serving Medicare and Medicaid beneficiaries are not required to provide basic services which are not compensated under these programs, nor to fix payments by community rating.

Employees Health Benefit Plans

Every employer of 25 or more persons is to include in health benefit plans offered to employees the option to enroll in health maintenance organizations which are providing services in the areas in which the employees reside.

Restrictive State Laws and Practices

State requirements which prevent an entity from functioning as a health maintenance organization (as defined in this legislation) shall not apply. Specifically, preempted restrictions are:

- Requirement of approval by a medical society of services furnished
- Requirement that physicians constitute all or a percentage of the governing body
- Requirement that all or a percentage of physicians be permitted to participate in the provision of services
- Certain requirements for insurers

- Prohibition of solicitation of members through advertising of services, charges or other nonprofessional aspects of an organization's operation

Quality Assurance

A new part is added to Title III of the Public Health Service Act: Part K—*Quality Assurance.*

The Secretary, through the Assistant Secretary of Health, is to conduct research and evaluation programs respecting the effectiveness, administration and enforcement of quality assurance programs.

The Secretary is also directed to make an annual report to Congress and the President on the quality of health care in the United States, the operation of quality assurance programs, and advances made through research and evaluation.

Other Studies and Reports

The Secretary is to contract with a nonprofit organization of recognized competence for the conduct of a general study in the area of quality assurance. The study is to include analysis of methodologies, the delineation of basic principles for quality assurance systems, the definition of need in the area of research and evaluation related to health care quality, and the provision of methods for quality assessment from the point of view of consumers. Interim and final reports of the study are to be submitted to the appropriate Congressional committees.

19. NATIONAL HEALTH PLANNING AND RESOURCES DEVELOPMENT ACT OF 1974*

"An Act to amend the Public Health Service Act to assure the development of a national health policy and of effective state and area health planning and resource development program, and for other purposes."

Two new titles, XV and XVI, were added to the Public Health Service Act. They superseded and greatly modified the previous programs established under sections 314a and 314b of Title III (Comprehensive Health Planning), Title VI (Hill-Burton) and Title IX (Regional Medical Programs). A brief summary of the major provisions follows.

*PL 93-641

Title XV—National Health Planning and Development

Part A—National Guidelines for Health Planning

The Secretary is to issue *national health policy planning* guidelines, formulated in consideration of stated *national health priorities.* A National Advisory Council on Health Planning and Development is established.

Part B—Health Systems Agencies

Provision is made for the establishment of *health service areas* and *health systems agencies* throughout the United States.

A health service area, to be designated by the state Governor, will in general have a population of 500,000 to 3,000,000, and have boundaries coordinated with those of Professional Standards Review Organizations and existing planning areas. Except under certain circumstances, each standard metropolitan statistical area is to be within the boundaries of one health service area.

A non-profit (health planning or development) corporation, public regional planning body, or unit of local government may apply for designation as a health systems agency. Each agency is to have appropriate staff and a governing body of which a majority are to be area residents and consumers.

The stated purposes of the agencies are: 1) improving the health of area residents, 2) increasing the accessibility, acceptability, continuity and quality of health services, and 3) restraining costs and preventing duplication of health services.

The functions of the agencies include the collection and analysis of data, establishment of *health systems plans* (HSP's) and *annual implementation plans* (AIP's), and the making of grants and contracts from an Area Health Services Development Fund to be established. They are to review and approve or disapprove the use of Federal funds in the area for health services or resources development; and periodically review all institutional health services for appropriateness; and annually recommend to the State agency [see Part C] projects for modernization, construction and conversion of medical facilities.

Planning grants will be made annually to each health service agency according to a per capita formula. The basic grant is to be the lesser of $0.50 per person in the area or $3,750,000.

Part C—State Health Planning and Development

The Secretary is to enter into agreements with the Governors of each State for the designation of a *State health planning and development* agency. If such an agreement is not in effect after four years, no funds may be made available under the Public Health Service Act, Community Mental Health Centers Act or the Comprehensive Alcoholic Abuse and Alcoholism Act for the development or support of health resources in the States. A Statewide Health Coordinating Council is also to be established.

The functions of the State agency are to: 1) conduct health planning for the State, 2) prepare (from the HSP's) and annually review a State health plan for submission to the Coordinating Council, 3) assist the council in review of the State medical facilities plan [see Title XVI] and other functions, 4) administer a *State certificate of need program*, 5) periodically review all institutional services in the State with regard to appropriateness.

The State Health Coordinating Council is to be appointed by the Governor, with a majority of the members to be appointed from among nominees from the health systems agencies.

The Council is to: 1) annually review and coordinate the HSP's and AIP's, 2) review annually the State health plan, 3) annually review the budgets of the health systems agencies, 4) review grant applications for Federal funds under the Public Health Service Act, Community Mental Health Centers Act or the Comprehensive Alcohol Abuse and Alcoholism Act. Disapprovals may be reviewed, at State request, by the Secretary.

Grants are to be made to the State agencies for up to 75% of their costs.

Grants may be made to (not more than six) State agencies for the purpose of demonstrating their effectiveness in regulating rates for the provision of health care.

The Secretary is to provide to health systems agencies and State agencies assistance (directly or through grants and contracts) and technical materials for the development of their health plans and methodologies.

A *national health planning* information center is to be established to support the health planning and resource development programs.

The Secretary is to develop uniform systems for calculating services costs, volumes, and rates to be charged, for cost accounting and for classifying health services institutions.

The Secretary is to assist by grants or contracts the development of *centers for health planning.*

Title XVI—Health Resources Development

Part A—Purpose, State Plan and Project Approval

The purpose of this title is to provide assistance for projects for modernization of medical facilities, construction of new outpatient facilities, construction of new inpatient facilities in areas of recent rapid population growth, and conversion of facilities for the provision of new health services, and for projects related to the elimination of safety hazards and the avoidance of noncompliance with licensure or accreditation standards.

The Secretary is to prescribe among other requirements the general manner in which the State Agency shall determine priorities for projects; general standards of construction and modernization; criteria for determining needs; and requirements whereby each State medical facilities plan is to provide for facilities adequate for all State residents and the furnishing of needed services for persons unable to pay therefor.

A *State medical facilities plan* must be submitted by the State Agency. The plan must, among other requirements, be approved by the Statewide Health Coordinating Council as consistent with the State health plan.

Project applications must, among other requirements, include reasonable assurances that the assisted facility will be made available to all persons in the area and that a reasonable volume of services will be made available to persons unable to pay therefor (subject to determination by the Secretary of financial feasibility). Each application is to be reviewed by the appropriate health systems agencies.

Part B—Allotments

Allotments are to be made to the States from appropriated funds on the basis of population, financial need, and need for medical facilities.

Requirements include the stipulation that not more than 20 percent of a State's allotment may be obligated for construction of new inpatient facilities and not less than 25 percent is to be obligated for outpatient facilities for medically underserved populations, including rural populations.

Part C—Loans and Loan Guarantees

Provision is made for a program of loans and loan guarantees for projects approved under Part A.

Part D—Project Grants

Provision is made for construction or modernization projects designed to eliminate or prevent safety hazards or to avoid non-compliance with State or voluntary licensure or accreditation standards. Such grants are to be made only to public or quasi-public entities. Twenty-two percent of the funds appropriated under Part A are to be made available for such projects.

Part E—General Provisions

General provisions related to judicial review of project disapprovals, recovery of funds, financial statements, definitions and technical assistance.

The *Federal share* of the costs of a grant-assisted project may be up to 66-2/3 percent (up to 100 percent in the case of an urban or rural poverty area).

Part F—Area Health Services
Development Funds

Funds are authorized to be appropriated from which the Secretary is to make each year a grant to each health systems agency for an *Area Health Services Development Fund* from which grants and contracts may be made. The amount of each agency grant is to be related to the population, average family income, and supply of health services in the area.

Transitional provisions include limited authorization for grants under section 314a, 314b and Title IX; such funds to be available up to three months after the designation of the State and area agencies established under this Act.

Administration

Health Resources Administration (Bureau of Health Planning and Resources Development)

Note

As of May 1976, 202 health service areas have been approved and 100 health systems agencies designated. Most of the latter are former comprehensive health planning ("314 b") agencies.

20. SUMMARY OF PUBLIC HEALTH SERVICE ACT TITLES

Title I   *Short Title and Definitions*

Title II   *Administration*

General Organisation of the Public Health Service and the Commisioned Corps

Title III   *General Powers and Duties of the Public Health Service*

    A. Research and Investigation
        Includes national health surveys and studies, public health traineeships and project grants, and health services for agricultural migrants
    B. Federal-State Cooperation
        Includes comprehensive public health services (section 314)
    C. Hospitals, Medical Examinations and Medical Care
    D. Lepers
    E. Narcotic Addicts and Other Drug Abuses
    F. Licensing—Biological Products and Clinical Laboratories and Control of Radiation
    G. Quarantine and Inspection
    H. Grants to Alaska for Mental Health (Repealed)
    I. National Library of Medicine
    J. Assistance to Medical Libraries
    K. Quality Assurance

Title IV   *National Research Institutes*

    A. National Cancer Institute
    B. National Heart Institute

C. National Institute of Dental Research

D. National Institute on Arthritis, Metabolism and Digestive Diseases; National Institute of Neurological Diseases and Stroke; and Other Institutes

E. National Institutes of Child Health and Human Development and of General Medical Sciences

F. National Eye Institute

G. National Institute of Mental Health

H. Administrative Provisions
Includes provisions relating to the director of the National Institutes of Health and the director of the National Cancer Institute

Title V   *Miscellaneous*

Title VI   *Assistance for Construction and Modernization of Hospitals and Other Medical Facilities*

A. Grants and Loans for Construction and Modernization of Hospitals and Other Medical Facilities

B. Loan Guarantees and Loans for Modernization and Construction of Hospitals and Other Medical Facilities

C. Construction or Modernization of Emergency Rooms

D. General

Title VII   *Health Research and Teaching Facilities and Training of Professional Health Personnel*

A. Grants for Construction of Health Research Facilities

B. Grants for Construction of Teaching Facilities for Medical, Dental and Other Health Personnel

C. Student Loans

D. Grants for Family Medicine, Training, Traineeships and Fellowships and Computer Technology Health Care Demonstration Programs

E. Grants and Contracts to Improve the Quality of Schools of Medicine, Osteopathy, Dentistry, Veterinary Medicine, Optometry, Pharmacy and Podiatry; Health Manpower Educational Initiative Awards

F. Scholarship Grants to Schools of Medicine, Osteopathy, Dentistry, Optometry, Podiatry, Pharmacy or Veterinary Medicine

          G. Training in the Allied Health Professions
          H. General Provisions

Title VIII   *Nurse Training*

          A. Grants for Expansion and Improvement of Nurse Training
          B. Assistance to Nursing Students
          C. General (National Advisory Council on Nurse Training; Review Committee)
          D. Scholarship Grants to Schools of Nursing

Title IX   *Education, Research, Training, and Demonstrations in the Fields of Heart Disease, Cancer, Stroke, Kidney Disease, and Other Related Diseases*

Title X   *Population Research and Voluntary Family Planning Programs*

Title XI   *Genetic Blood Disorders and Sudden Infant Death Syndrome*

          A. Sickle Cell Anemia Programs
          B. Cooley's Anemia Programs
          C. Sudden Infant Death Syndrome
          D. Hemophilia Programs

Title XII   *Emergency Medical Services Systems*

Title XIII   *Health Maintenance Organizations*

Title XIV   *Safety of Public Water Systems**

Title XV   *National Health Planning and Development*

          A. National Guidelines for Health Planning
          B. Health Systems Agencies
          C. State Health Planning and Development
          D. General Provisions
             Includes provisions for the development of centers for health planning

Title XVI   *Health Resources Development*

          A. Purpose, State Plan and Project Approval
          B. Allotments
          C. Loans and Loan Guarantees

*PL 93-523, Safe Drinking Water Act, administered by the Environmental Protection Agency.

D. Project Grants
E. General Provisions
F. Area Health Services Development Funds

21. MENTAL RETARDATION FACILITIES AND COMMUNITY MENTAL HEALTH CENTERS CONSTRUCTION ACT OF 1963

"An Act to provide assistance in combating mental retardation through grants for construction of research centers and grants for facilities for the mentally retarded and assistance in improving mental health through grants for construction of community mental health centers, and for other purposes."

Background

Congressional interest in the problem of mental health was first expressed in the *Mental Health Act of 1946* which specifically provided for the inclusion of mental health problems in the grant-in-aid programs of the Public Health Service Act and established the National Institute of Mental Health patterned after the National Cancer Institute. The *Mental Health Study Act of 1955* authorized grants to facilitate a program of research into resources and methods for care of the mentally ill,[94] and in 1956 the *Health Amendments Act* added special project grants particularly directed to the problems of state mental hospitals. Legislation addressed to the problem of mental retardation was added in 1963 in the *Maternal and Child Health and Mental Retardation Planning Amendments.*[95]

Summary of Major Provisions

Title I. Construction of Research Centers and Facilities for the Mentally Retarded—"Mental Retardation Facilities Construction Act"

Part A. Grants for Construction of Centers for Research on Mental Retardation and Related Aspects of Human Development

Amends Title VII of the Public Health Service Act to authorize

[94] The resultant Joint Commission on Mental Illness and Health published a final report, *Action for Mental Health*, in 1961.

[95] See p. 145

grants to assist in the construction of facilities for research relating to mental retardation.[95] Federal participation: up to 75 percent.

Part B. Project Grants for Construction of University Affiliated Facilities for the Mentally Retarded

Grants for the construction of university-affiliated facilities providing a full range of inpatient and outpatient services; for demonstrating specialized services for the mentally retarded; or for clinical training of physicians and other specialized personnel. Federal participation: up to 75 percent.

Part C. Grants for the Construction of Facilities for the Mentally Retarded

Grants to the states for the construction of community facilities for the mentally retarded; patterned after the Hill-Burton program. Federal share: 33-1/3 to 66-2/3 percent.

Title II. Construction of Community Mental Health Centers—"Community Mental Health Centers Act"

Grants to the states for construction of community mental health centers, also generally patterned after the Hill-Burton Program. Federal share: 33-1/3 to 66-2/3 percent.

Title III. Training of Teachers of Mentally Retarded and Other Handicapped Children

Extends and strengthens existing programs for training teachers of mentally retarded and deaf children,[97] and expands them to include the training of teachers of other handicapped children.

Title IV. General

Definitions include:

Community Mental Health Center—A facility providing services for the prevention or diagnosis of mental illness, or care and treatment of mentally ill patients, or rehabilitation of such persons, which services are provided principally for persons residing in a particular community or communities in or near which the facility is situated.

[96] Under the program of construction grants established by the Health Research Facilities Act of 1956.

[97] Legislation (PL 85-929, 1958) authorizing grants to educational institutions and agencies for training teachers of mentally retarded children.

Construction—Construction of new buildings, expansion, remodeling and alteration of existing buildings, and initial equipment for any such buildings.

Amendments to the Mental Retardation and Community Mental Health Centers Legislation

The 1965 amendments to this legislation included provisions for grants to assist in meeting the initial cost of professional and technical personnel for community mental health centers (30–75 percent), and grants to institutions of higher education for construction of facilities for research in the field of education of handicapped children.

The *Mental Health Amendments of 1967* extended the program of grants for construction and initial staffing of community mental health centers and amended the term "construction" to include acquisition of existing buildings. The *Mental Retardation Amendments of 1967* extended the program of construction grants for university affiliated and community facilities for the mentally retarded, and established a program of initial staffing grants analogous to those for community mental health centers. A new title was added: Title V— "Training of Physical Educators and Recreation Personnel for Mentally Retarded and Other Handicapped Children." This authorized grants to educational institutions for the training of such personnel and for related research and demonstration projects.

The Alcoholic and Narcotic Addict Rehabilitation Amendments of 1968[98] added new provisions to the Community Mental Health Centers Act, relating to alcoholism and narcotic addiction: grants for construction and initial staffing of facilities for the treatment and rehabilitation of alcoholics[99] and narcotic addicts and grants for special training programs and evaluation studies relating to narcotic addiction services.

The Community Mental Health Centers Amendments of 1970 extended the program of construction grants and changed the definition of construction to include the acquisition of land. The dura-

[98] A section of the Public Health Service Amendments of 1968 which also amended the Regional Medical Programs and the Hill-Burton and Migratory Workers Programs.

[99] These facilities to be associated with other mental health services program, including community mental health centers.

tion of initial staffing grants was lengthened to eight years and, for centers in poverty areas, the grant ceiling was increased to 70-90 percent. Provision was also made for centers in poverty areas to begin operation (for 18 months) without furnishing all the "essential" components of comprehensive mental health services.[100] Additionally, grants were authorized to local agencies for development of community mental health services in rural or urban poverty areas.

The program of grants for facilities and services for alcoholics and narcotic addicts was also extended,[101] the duration of the staffing grants lengthened, and the grant ceiling increased, for centers in poverty areas. Special project grants were authorized for training, surveys, treatment and rehabilitation projects.

The Community Mental Health Centers Act was further amended by the addition of a part on Mental Health of Children. This authorized grants for construction of facilities[102] for the mental health of children, the cost of professional and technical personnel for new facilities or new services, and for training and program evaluation.

The *Comprehensive Drug Abuse Prevention and Control Act of 1970*[103] included provisions broadening the scope of narcotic addiction programs to include drug abuse and drug dependence, authorized grants for programs and activities related to drug education and special project grants for drug abuse and addiction treatment and rehabilitation. Provisions of the *Comprehensive Alcohol Abuse and Alcoholism Prevention, Treatment and Rehabilitation Act of 1970* added to the Community Mental Health Centers Act provisions for project grants and contracts in the area of prevention and treatment of alcohol abuse and alcoholism.[104]

[100] As specified in regulations, these services are:

"1. Inpatient services
2. Outpatient services
3. Partial hospitalization services—must include at least day care service
4. Emergency services provided 24 hours per day . . .
5. Consultation and education services [for] community agencies and professional personnel."

[101] The alcoholism section of this program had not yet been implemented.

[102] Associated with a community mental health center or other appropriate facility.

[103] Title II of this legislation is named the *Controlled Substances Act*. It contains provisions for drug abuse related control and enforcement by the Department of Justice.

[104] This comprehensive alcoholism act also (1) established the National Institute on Alcohol Abuse and Alcoholism in the National Institute of Mental Health and a national Advisory Council on Alcohol Abuse and Alcoholism, (2) directed the

The Developmental Disabilities Services and Facilities Construc-tion Amendments of 1970 extended the mental retardation programs and broadened the language of the legislation to include other neu-rological handicapping conditions. The *Developmentally Disabled Assistance and Bill of Rights Act* (1975) extended and further re-vised these programs.

The *Community Mental Health Centers Amendments of 1975* extended and revised the community mental health centers program. Additions included requirements that centers include programs of specialized services for children and the elderly, and provisions for governing bodies or advisory committees made up of area residents.

22. ECONOMIC OPPORTUNITY ACT OF 1964—
"Anti-Poverty Program"

"An Act to mobilize the human and financial resources of the Nation to combat poverty in the United States."

Title I.   *Work Training and Work Study Programs*

    A. Establishes the Job Corps (conservation camps and residential training centers).

    B. Work-training programs for unemployed youths and young adults (Neighborhood Youth Corps).

    C. Work-study programs in colleges and universities for students from low income families

Title II.   *Urban and Rural Community Action Programs*

    A. Grants for antipoverty programs to be planned and carried out at the community level. Programs are to be administered by the communities and are to mobilize all available resources and facilities in a coordinated attack on poverty.

    B. Grants to the states for basic adult education pro-grams.

    C. Voluntary assistance program for needy children (information and coordination office).

Title III.   *Antipoverty Programs in Rural Areas*

    A. Loans to low income rural families.

Civil Service Commission to develop appropriate prevention, treatment, and re-habilitation programs for Federal employees, and (3) authorized formula grants to the states for projects related to prevention, treatment and rehabilitation.

B.   Assistance for housing, sanitation, education, and child care programs for migrant farm workers.

C.   Indemnity payments to farmers for pesticide-contaminated milk.

Title IV.   *Assistance to Small Business Concerns*

Loans and management training for small businesses.

Title V.   *Work Experience Programs*

Grants for experimental and demonstration work experience and training programs for unemployed persons on public assistance.

Title VI.   *Administration and Coordination*

Establishes the Office of Economic Opportunity and provides for administration of the Act. Authorizes the program *Volunteers in Service to America* (VISTA).

Title VII.   *Exemption of Income for Public Assistance Purposes*

Exemption of part or all of earnings under the Economic Opportunity Act from consideration as income or resources of public assistance recipients.

Office of Economic Opportunity (Executive Office of the President)

- Direct responsibility for the *Job Corps, community action programs, VISTA*, and the programs for migrant farm workers;
- Indirect (delegated) responsibility for the work study, adult education and work experience programs (HEW); the work training programs (Department of Labor); the special rural programs (Department of Agriculture); and the small business programs (Small Business Administration);
- Coordination of the poverty-related programs of all federal agencies.

Community Action Programs

The legislation defines a community action program eligible for federal assistance as one which:

"Mobilizes and utilizes resources, public or private . . . in an attack on poverty;

Provides services, assistance and other activities [which] give promise of progress toward the elimination of poverty or a cause or causes of poverty ... ;

Is developed, conducted and administered with the *maximum feasible participation of residents of the areas and members of the groups served*; and

Is conducted, administered or coordinated by a public or nonprofit agency, or combination thereof."

Community action programs could be conducted in such fields as employment, job training and counseling, health, vocational rehabilitation, housing, home management, welfare, and special remedial and other noncurricular educational assistance.

Among the many programs which were developed under the community action provisions, and which were given statutory recognition in amendments to this Title, are the OEO neighborhood health centers (comprehensive health services programs), the Head Start child development programs, the legal services programs and the family planning and drug rehabilitation programs.

The Economic Opportunity Act, often controversial, has been much amended, and many administrative changes have been made. Notably, the Job Corps and Neighborhood Youth Corps are now administered by the Department of Labor, the VISTA program has been combined with the Peace Corps in a new ACTION agency, the Head Start program has been placed in HEW's Office of Child Development, and the neighborhood health centers have been transferred to the Public Health Service.

In 1975, under the *Headstart, Economic Opportunity and Community Partnership Act*, the Office of Economic Opportunity was abolished and replaced by the independent *Community Services Administration* which· now administers the community action programs.[105]

23. A NOTE TO THE READER

Many details of the book will be altered by the swift pace of changing events.

---

[105] A nonprofit *Legal Services Corporation* for the legal assistance programs had been previously established by the Legal Services Corporation Act of 1974.

This is particularly true of these sections dealing with federal legislation and the organization of federal agencies.

In the case of Congressional activity this problem can be dealt with without undue difficulty if the interested reader will, once having acquired a basic understanding of the progression of the laws, develop a systematic approach to keeping abreast of developments. One method would be the regular scanning of the *Congressional Quarterly* or the *U.S. Code Congressional and Administrative News.* Systematic review of one of the many Washington newsletters would also be useful. Examples of these are the *Washington Report on Medicine and Health* and the letters published by the various interested associations, such as the American Public Health Association, the American Public Welfare Association, and the Association of American Medical Colleges. A regular *Memorandum* published by the Special Committee on Aging, United States Senate, is good for matters affecting the elderly, including Social Security amendments.

I have yet to find a really good way to keep up with the various activities and reorganizations of the federal agencies. The above newsletters are helpful. Direct inquiries to the agency of interest will elicit information, although the substantive quality varies widely. Some put out regular newsletters.

Significant reorganizations and all administrative regulations are published in the *Federal Register.* Those who are involved with federal programs usually take care to watch for these.

Obtaining Documents

Single copies of bills, laws, committee hearings and reports can usually be obtained from the House or Senate Document Room, Washington, D.C.; zip codes 20515 and 20510, respectively. (Enclose a self-addressed label.) These can often also be obtained from the Congressional Committees or from individual Congressmen and Senators.

Similarly, single copies of many reports and publications can be obtained from the relevant agencies.

The U.S. Government Printing Office publishes a monthly catalog of published documents which are for sale at usually reasonable prices.

References

Congressional Quarterly and Almanac, (Washington, D.C.: Congressional Quarterly, Inc.) Weekly summary and commentary on Congressional activities.

U.S. Code Congressional and Administrative News, (St. Paul, Minnesota: West Publishing Co.) Monthly Congressional summary with texts of newly passed laws and related committee reports.

Washington Report on Medicine and Health, (Washington, D.C.: McGraw-Hill, Inc.) A weekly commentary on federal events, particularly legislative

Chapter 5

State and Local Health Activities

In general, the responsibility for the general public health and welfare resides with the states.[1]

The many state activities related to health include:

- Traditional public health functions related to the promotion of health and the prevention of disease, such as communicable disease control, sanitation and the assurance of the quality of water and food supplies.
- Provision of direct institutional services for long-term conditions such as tuberculosis, mental illness, mental retardation, and chronic disease. Such services are generally beyond the capacity of the private or public sectors of the local communities.
- Regulatory Functions. These include the licensing of health professionals and of health facilities; the regulation, under the insurance laws, of heath insurance companies and organizations; and the establishment of health and safety codes for housing, institutions and industry. Recent developments in many states have been the enactment of "certificate of need" legislation controlling the construction and establishment of health facilities and programs, and the establishment of rate-setting bodies.
- Planning Functions. The states participate in health planning activities through state health planning agencies.
- Educational Functions. There are many programs for health man-

[1] In theory, all governmental authority resides in the states, except as delegated by them to the federal government, under the Constitution or to local jurisdictions, by legislation.

power education and training in the state colleges, universities, and other institutions. These include medicine, nursing, pharmacy, and many others.

- Administration of federally aided programs. Most federal grant-in-aid programs are administered by the cooperating state agencies. (Examples are the Hill-Burton, Medicaid, community mental health centers, and vocational rehabilitation programs.) Certain aspects of other programs are also handled by state agencies; (for example, the surveying and certification of institutional providers of services under Medicare).

Health-related services in the states, and as delegated to the counties, cities, and towns, are provided by a complex and ever-changing variety of agencies and organizations in patterns which differ from state to state. Many of them are lodged in *departments of public health*. Many are typically lodged elsewhere. For example, there is often a separate state department of mental health; licensing of health manpower may be a responsibility of departments of education; vocational rehabilitation programs are often administered by separate agencies; occupational health (industrial hygiene) is usually lodged in state departments of labor; and school health is commonly the responsibility of boards of education. Recently, several states have placed environmental control programs in separate agencies.

Public Health Departments

The traditional "basic six"[2] functions of public health agencies are:

1. Collection of *vital statistics* of births, deaths, and reportable diseases
2. Control of communicable diseases, including tuberculosis and venereal diseases
3. Environmental sanitation, including water quality and supervision of foods and eating places
4. Public health laboratory services
5. Maternal and child health, including school health
6. Health education

Notable additions to the list in recent years have been activities directed to problems such as *nutrition, chronic disease, dental health, radiological control, air quality control, alcohol and drug abuse* and *family planning.*

---

[2] As set forth in the report *Local Health Units for the Nation* by Haven Emerson, The Commonwealth Fund, 1945.

Health agencies, at various levels, have traditionally been organized in appropriate divisions and bureaus to carry out these functions which are largely concerned with the prevention of disease and disability.

In recent years there has been a great increase in health planning, regulatory, standard-setting, and monitoring functions, especially with regard to health care institutions such as hospitals and nursing homes. These activities were originally greatly stimulated by the federal Hill-Burton legislation directed to hospital planning and construction and more recently by provision of the Medicare-Medicaid and Comprehensive Health Planning laws. These trends have been augmented by the rapid development of "certificate of need" legislation by the states. Many of these functions have been placed in health agencies but many have been placed in other agencies, the pattern again varying from state to state.

Many health departments have also become increasingly concerned with the problems of the provision of direct medical care services, especially to low income populations.

State Health Departments

In most of the states, primary responsibility for public health is lodged in a separate state department of health.[3] There is also usually a *Board of Health*, with varying advisory, policy and administrative functions, with members generally appointed by the governor. The chief executive officer (health officer, director, commissioner) is also usually appointed by the governor or by the board.

State departments of health delegate most direct services to the local departments[4] providing them general liaison, consultation, and special services as needed. The state agencies usually retain certain statewide regulatory and planning functions, such as professional and health facilities licensure and statewide comprehensive health planning.[5]

---

[3] In some states, the health agency is combined with one or more other agencies, most often the department of public welfare (now commonly termed "Social Services").

[4] A notable exception being the operation of such facilities as chronic disease and tuberculosis hospitals.

[5] The State comprehensive health planning "A" agencies were established in response to 1966 federal legislation (see p. 000) and were variously lodged in state health departments, in interdepartmental commissions, or in governors' executive offices. As of this writing, they are being reorganized as or replaced by *state health planning and development agencies* under 1974 federal legislation (see p. 187).

Local Health Departments

With a few exceptions, mostly in some rural western counties,[6] all areas of the United States are served by local health units—county, city, town, or (a few instances) combined city and county.[7] The number and scope of services provided vary greatly.

There are local *boards of health* with members appointed by elected officials—county commissioners or supervisors, mayors, or town selectmen. The health officer is typically appointed by the board generally in accordance with qualifications set by the state department of health.[8]

Staff of a local health unit will include as a minimum the health officer, one or more public health nurses, and one or more sanitary engineers or sanitarians. With increasing scope of responsibilities, the number and types of professional and technical staff will increase commensurately and may include dentists, social workers, health educators, nutritionists, epidemiologists, special laboratory personnel, and many others.

Where many and complex services are provided, the health officer will serve as director or commissioner of an organized department of health with appropriate divisions; here the basic unit for provision of direct services to the population is usually the *health center*. Large health departments may be partially decentralized, with district health officers and centers.

The health center will house services such as maternity and family planning clinics, well baby and child health clinics, tuberculosis and venereal disease units, dental clinics (usually for children), nutrition and health education services, and field personnel for environmental health programs. Some health centers in low income communities have in recent years been providing treatment as well as preventive services for children, usually in cooperation with a local hospital; health centers have also been the base for some of the federally funded health care programs and neighborhood health centers.

"Umbrella Agencies"

In recent years a number of state and local jurisdictions have attempted to consolidate and streamline health and welfare services

[6] But also in parts of New York State and all of Rhode Island.

[7] Where there is no local health unit, services are provided by regional or district offices of the state health department.

[8] Generally, though not invariably, the health officer is a physician.

by combining related departments and agencies into one overall administrative structure. These "umbrella agencies" or "super agencies" have involved varying combinations of departments of health, hospitals,[9] mental health, public welfare, rehabilitation, youth services, and others. Examples of such amalgamations are the North Carolina Department of Human Resources, the Suffolk County (New York) Department of Health Services, and the New York City Health Services Administration.

Reference

Public Health Administration and Practice, Sixth Edition, John J. Hanlon (Saint Louis: The C.V. Mosby Company, 1974).

[9] In some jurisdictions which maintain county or municipal hospitals.

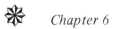 *Chapter 6*

Ambulatory Care
(Non-Institutional Care)

Strictly speaking, the term *ambulatory care* refers to care rendered to patients who come to physicians' offices, outpatient departments, and health centers. However, it often includes by extension other hospital-related, non-inpatient components of care such as emergency and home care services. The term is also often used with the same connotation as *community medicine*.

This field is complex and many of its aspects are rapidly changing in concept and terminology. The following are brief descriptions of components which are of particular importance or current interest.

Forms of Physician Practice

Solo Practice.[1] Independent practice by a physician usually using his own facilities and equipment, but sometimes sharing these with one or more other physicians. A formal arrangement for using common facilities is often termed an *association*.

Partnership. A legal agreement between two or more physicians to share income and assets in an unincorporated business, with each partner legally the agent of the other. Many group practices are in

[1] Legally, a solo practitioner is a *sole proprietor*—a one-man owner of an unincorporated business.

209

fact partnerships, although they frequently include salaried physicians among their staff.

Group Practice. There is no one generally accepted definition of group practice, but the common denominator is a voluntary association of three or more physicians in medical practice who use common facilities and share income in a designated way.

The American Medical Association defines a group practice as "the application of medical services by three or more physicians formally organized to provide medical care, consultation, diagnosis and/or treatment through the joint use of equipment and personnel, and with the income from medical practice distributed in accordance with methods previously determined by members of the group."

Groups so defined consist of three categories:

1. Single specialty groups
2. General practice groups
3. Multi-specialty groups (providing services in at least two specialties)

Other definitions specify that services include those of more than one specialty.

The first group practice, a multispecialty group, was the well-known Mayo Clinic, established in Rochester, Minnesota in the decade prior to 1900. Group practices began to develop in significant numbers in the 1920s, particularly in the West and Midwest, but their growth was relatively slow, with further relative increases after World War II. In 1969 there were upward of 6,000 group practices, involving about 40,000 physicians. Of these, about half were single specialty groups.[2]

Many of the larger group practices are associated with prepayment plans; among these are the Permanente groups (Kaiser Foundation Health Plan) and the HIP groups (Health Insurance Plan of Greater New York, New York City).

Associations

American Group Practice Association[3]

[2] For an extensive survey of groups, see: C. Todd and M.E. McNamara, *Medical Groups in the U.S. 1969*, Special Statistical Series, American Medical Association, 1971.

[3] Formerly American Association of Medical Clinics.

Medical Group Management Association[4]
Group Health Association of America[5]

Professional Corporation. A legal entity which is distinct from its members. There is limited liability for corporate debts, but a physician member remains liable for his own negligent acts. Most states now permit the establishment of professional corporations, which carry certain tax advantages and other benefits. Solo practitioners as well as groups of physicians may incorporate.[6]

Centers, Programs and Agencies

Outpatient Department. In the past often termed "dispensary,"[7] now apt to be called an ambulatory care service. A hospital department where persons not requiring hospitalization may receive care; it is usually distinguished from the *emergency room*, although persons with non-urgent problems are often also seen in the latter area, especially during hours when the outpatient unit is not open. It is commonly referred to as the *clinic*, as are its component units, i.e., medical clinic, surgical clinic. (This term is also often used for large group practices, such as the Mayo Clinic.)

Population served is generally a medically indigent one, although middle income levels may be served, especially at university teaching hospitals, and special consultation mechanisms may be available for referring physicians.

Patients are usually seen by house staff (interns and residents) or unpaid attending physicians (voluntary staff).

Increasingly, private patients may be seen by physicians who have offices at the hospital under rental or other arrangements. This is usually distinguished from the general Outpatient Department by a term such as "private ambulatory service."

[4] Formerly National Association of Clinic Managers.

[5] Prepaid health plans.

[6] A series of court decisions led the Internal Revenue Service in 1969 to give corporate tax status to professional corporations; this in turn has resulted in a significant increase in their number.

[7] Dispensaries were originally independent charitable entities for the treatment of sick poor. They developed in parallel with hospitals and were ultimately displaced by hospital outpatient departments.

Health Center. This term has been used to refer to the locus of a wide variety of health care and related activities, and generally implies services to a specific local area, district, or neighborhood. It commonly means a unit of a city or county health department, housing services such as well child and prenatal clinics, and venereal disease and tuberculosis control and treatment units; emphasis is on preventive services.

Neighborhood Health Center. A health center whose purpose is to provide a program of comprehensive health services to a defined local area, often with related social services, and generally with some degree, often considerable, of involvement and participation of members of the local community. The use of non-traditional personnel such as family health workers[8] and emphasis on "health care teams" are characteristic of these centers.

Most were developed in the 1960s with federal funding under legislation such as the Economic Opportunity Act,[9] Title V of the Social Security Act,[10] and Model Cities. Many are sponsored by local health departments. Some centers are independent but most have some degree of hospital affiliation and may be termed, from the hospital viewpoint, *satellite centers*. A "back-up" hospital is one which provides specialized services and hospital admissions for a neighborhood health center.

Analogous programs are the rural health centers developed under federal financing for migrant health and Appalachian development, as well as under the Economic Opportunity Act.

Mental Health Center (Community Mental Health Center). A center for the provision of comprehensive mental health services, usually to a defined geographical "catchment" area. It emphasizes the provision of a wide range of mental health services in the com-

---

[8] The family health worker is a health occupation developed at the Dr. Martin Luther King, Jr. Health Center in New York City and described by Harold B. Wise. It is representative of a cadre of newly trained, previously unskilled workers, typically recruited from the communities served. They carry out a variety of delegated nursing, health education, social service and social advocacy functions in health centers and the community. Terminology is diverse and includes community health aides, health guides, neighborhood aides, neighborhood health agents and "out-reach" workers.

[9] Funded the OEO (Office of Economic Opportunity) neighborhood health centers, which were the origins of the current neighborhood health center movement.

[10] Maternity and Infant Care, Children and Youth Projects.

munity as opposed to the more traditional emphasis of long-term hospitalization of the mentally ill. As defined in federal regulations[11] for purposes of eligibility for funding support, a community health center is one which provides a spectrum of services including, in addition to inpatient services available to the community, outpatient, day care and 24-hour emergency services, and consultation and educational services for community agencies and professional personnel. A community mental health center need not be a physical entity; it can actually be a network of coordinated services. Teams are also emphasized here, as well as short term and "crisis intervention" approaches to treatment. Much use is also made of community workers trained as mental health aides.

Drug Rehabilitation Programs. Programs for rehabilitation of drug abusers are of two major types: *Methadone maintenance;* hospital-related programs for heroin addicts based on the long-term use of methadone as a heroin substitute, supplemented in varying degrees by other rehabilitative services; and *Self-help:* community-based programs, some residential, which emphasize drug-free, group-oriented approaches; the term also often includes a wide spectrum of counseling and "hot-line" services.

"Free Clinics." Neighborhood clinics which provide medical services in relatively informal settings and styles to, generally, students, transient youth, and minority groups. Care is given at no or nominal charge by predominantly volunteer staffs. The first such clinic is considered to be the Haight-Ashbury Free Clinic, organized in San Francisco in the summer of 1967 by David Smith.

Short Stay Surgical Center ("Surgicenter"). An independent, usually proprietary, facility for surgical procedures which do not require overnight hospitalization. The principal rationale for the center is the reduction in costs compared with such hospitalization. The best known is the Surgicenter in Phoenix, established in 1970 by two anesthesiologists, John Ford and Wallace Reid.

Visiting Nurse Association (Visiting Nurse Service). A voluntary agency which provides nursing services in the home, including health supervision, education, and counseling; bedside care, and the carrying out of physicians' orders. They are staffed by public health nurses and often by other personnel such as physiotherapists, speech therapists and specially trained *home health aides.*

[11] Under the Community Mental Health Centers Act, 1963.

These agencies had their origin in the visiting or "district" nursing provided to sick poor in their homes by voluntary agencies, such as the New York City Mission, in the 1870s. The first visiting nurse associations were established in Buffalo, Boston and Philadelphia in 1886–87.

"Combined Agency."   A nursing agency jointly staffed by nurses from both voluntary (i.e., Visiting Nurse Association) and "official" agencies (i.e., city or county health department).

Home Care Program.   An organized program, hospital- or community-based, for the provision of a spectrum of medical services, equipment, and supplies to patients in their homes, generally patients with chronic illness. Community-based programs usually supplement the services of private practitioners; hospital-based programs may provide physician services. The earliest home care program, and still among the best known, was established in 1947 at Montefiore Hospital in New York City.

Home Health Agency.   A term defined in federal legislation (see p. 256) referring to an agency authorized to receive payment under federal programs (Medicare, Medicaid) for services provided in the home. Includes visiting nurse associations and home care programs.

Special Ambulatory Care Personnel

Public Health Nurse (Community Health Nurse).[12]   A public health nurse generally works in the community and is concerned with the health of groups and of persons in their usual environment such as home, school, or work. These nurses are most often based in health departments ("official agencies"), schools, or voluntary agencies such as visiting nurse associations. They traditionally function relatively independently and tend to be especially oriented toward the community, the family and the promotion of health and normal development. The nursing staffs of neighborhood health centers often include public health nurses.

Training includes experience in a community agency, either during a baccalaureate nursing program (as field experience) or after graduation from nursing school. Advanced training formerly ob-

---

[12] See Hanlon, John J., *Public Health Administration and Practice* (Reference, p. 207) for a good discussion of public health nursing.

tained by special courses granting a certificate is now obtained via master's degree programs.

Pediatric Nurse Practitioner.[13]   A pediatric nurse practitioner is a registered nurse who has been trained, in a program of four months' (or more) duration, to assume an expanded role in the care of children. This includes comprehensive well child care and the appraisal and management of certain conditions of the acute or chronically ill child. The first formal training program was developed in 1967 by Henry K. Silver and Loretta C. Ford at the Schools of Medicine and Nursing of the University of Colorado.

Other Practitioners.   More recently, training programs have been developed for "adult (medical) nurse practitioners" and "family nurse practitioners."

Legal Recognition.   The activities of nurse practitioners are generally considered as aspects of nursing practice, and specific new regulatory legislation has not been pursued. However, in the setting of the general trend toward expanded nursing roles many states have in the past few years amended their nursing practice acts to broaden the definition of nursing practice, and some amendments have included language directed to practitioners.

"Physician Extenders."   The general concept of "physician extenders" and "assistants for the physician" has attracted wide recent interest in the context of debate, discussion, and program development related to the "health manpower crisis" and the use of "allied health manpower." Terminology, goals, and programs are rapidly changing, and the following few descriptions merely illustrate some of the current trends.

Physician's Assistant (PA).[14]   A physician's assistant is trained to perform a variety of routine and delegated patient services under the supervision or direction of a physician. The first formal training program was established at Duke University in 1966 by Eugene A. Stead. The program comprises nine months' formal instruction and 15 months in clinical rotations, a format which is characteristic of many subsequent programs.

---

[13] Now often termed *Pediatric Nurse Associate.*

[14] Now sometimes termed *Physician's Associate.*

MEDEX.[15]   MEDEX programs are physician assistant programs which were developed specifically for former medical corpsmen with independent duty experience. Their purpose was to train extensions for physicians, especially for general practitioners in rural areas. (Most Medex have been trained to work with specific physicians). The first such program was begun in 1969 by Richard A. Smith at the University of Washington, in cooperation with the Washington State Medical Association. The programs generally consist of three months of university training and twelve months of preceptorship.

Child Health Associate.   This program was begun in 1969 at the University of Colorado for training child care professionals capable of handling a broad variety of non-life-threatening pediatric problems. This is a five-year program leading to a Bachelor of Science degree. (Two years undergraduate, two years at the medical center, one year of internship.)

Nurse practitioners (see above) are sometimes considered in the physician extender category.

Certification.   The National Board of Medical Examiners has developed in collaboration with the AMA's Council on Health Manpower a national certification examination for physician's assistants. The first such examination was given in December 1973. The program is now being administered by the newly formed *National Commission on Certification of Physician's Assistants.*

Legal Recognition.   The question of legal recognition of assistants to physicians has become an important and controversial one. A majority of states have passed relevant statutes, generally as amendments to medical practice acts. The earliest were those of California (for physician's assistants) and Colorado (for child health associates). Such statutes variably make explicit the authority of the physician to delegate functions, or provide for specific regulation by bodies such as the boards of medical examiners or registration.[16]

---

[15] From the French, "Médecin extension."

[16] A good discussion of the question of the legal regulation of both nurses and physician extenders may be found in *The Physician's Assistant Today and Tomorrow.* Alfred M. Sadler, Jr., Blair L. Sadler, and Ann A. Bliss: Chapter Four, "Where the Law Intervenes." (Cambridge: Ballinger Publishing Company, 1975).

Special Terms

"**Comprehensive Care.**" A system which provides a wide variety of health care services, with the implication that these will be coordinated, under the overall direction of a responsible physician or "team" of professionals, and with appropriate attention to preventive and rehabilitative services and socioeconomic factors.

"**Primary Care.**" A term, not yet well-defined, which has gained wide currency since the term *primary physician* was proposed in the report of the Citizens' Commission on Graduate Education in 1966.[17] Its meaning varies from that of "first contact" care (often with the implication of care simple to render, or of evaluation/referral) to that of broad, continuing responsibility for care of individuals or families; it is often used synonymously with family medicine, family practice, or general practice. It is also often used to denote care rendered by internists and pediatricians.

Triage.[18] This term is now commonly being used to describe the sorting out or screening of patients seeking care, to determine which service is initially required, and with what priority. A patient coming to a facility for care may be seen in a "triage," "screening" or "walk-in" clinic. Here it will be determined, possibly by a "triage nurse," whether, for example, the patient has a medical or surgical problem or requires some non-physician service such as social service consultation. Such rapid assessment units may merely refer patients to the most appropriate treatment service, or may also give treatment for minor problems.

Appointment System. The arrangement whereby a patient is given a definite time and date for a visit. *Block appointments* are those given for the same time to all patients, i.e., the beginning of a session. *Staggered appointments* are those given for a specific time during a session. These are also referred to as "wave" and "stream" systems. "*Walk-in*" refers to a patient who comes in for care without an appointment.

[17] *The Graduate Education of Physicians,* popularly known as the "Millis Report" after the Commission chairman, John S. Millis. The term was used to denote a physician who would be specially trained to provide comprehensive, continuing, health care. It is now often used as a generic term to refer to general or family practitioners, internists and pediatricians.

[18] From the French, "selecting, sifting," originally applied medically to the sorting of battle casualties.

Screening, Multi-Phasic Screening. Frequently an adjunct of ambulatory care programs; a system whereby a variety of routine tests are performed for the purpose of early disease detection.

Automated Multi-Phasic Health Testing (AMHT). A highly organized system of health testing which includes the use of automated equipment and data processing techniques.

Selected Readings

The Pediatric Nurse Practitioner Program: Expanding the Role of the Nurse to Provide Increased Health Care for Children, Henry K. Silver, Loretta C. Ford and Lewis R. Day, Journal of the American Medical Association, 204:298, 1968.

The Law and the Expanded Nursing Role, Bonnie Bullough, *Journal of the American Public Health Association,* 66:249, 1976.

Conserving Costly Talents—Providing Physicians New Assistants, Eugene A. Stead, Journal of the American Medical Association, 198:1108, 1966.

MEDEX, Richard A. Smith, Journal of the American Medical Association, 211:1843, 1970.

The Family Health Worker, Harold B. Wise, E. Fuller Torrey, Adrienne McDade, Gloria Perry and Harriet Bograd, American Journal of Public Health, 58:1828, 1968.

✳ *Chapter 7*

Voluntary Agencies

There is a wide variety of nonprofit organizations which are supported in whole or in part by private contributions and whose activities are directed to specific or general health or social welfare problems. They have been termed *voluntary agencies*, as distinct from "official" or governmental agencies.

Typically, voluntary agencies have been developed by private citizen groups, have predominantly lay boards and professional staff. Many are national bodies with local chapters and affiliates.

Examples are the American Cancer Society, American Heart Association, National Tuberculosis and Respiratory Disease Association,[1] and the National Association for Mental Health.

The activities of voluntary agencies are, in general, public education and support of studies, research, and often training in areas of their specific concern. Some also provide direct services (such as the family planning clinics of the Planned Parenthood Federation). Others, usually community based, are organized primarily for direct service; examples of these are family service agencies which provide counseling and other social services, and visiting nurse associations.

The American National Red Cross is unique in being a quasi-offi-

---

[1] This is the oldest voluntary health agency, with origins in the Anti-Tuberculosis Society of Philadelphia (1892) and the National Association for the Study and Prevention of Tuberculosis (1904). It was recently renamed the American Lung Association.

cial agency, chartered by Congress, and serving as the designated U.S. agency in national and international disaster relief.

There is also a variety of coordinating councils and agencies in which a number of organizations are loosely joined for planning, coordination, mutual education or fund raising purposes. Among these are the local community councils, united funds and community chests, and nationally, the National Health Council.

Philanthropic foundations have generally been established by single donors. Some provide support for relatively large research and demonstration programs and educational facilities. Foundations active in the health field include the Commonwealth Fund, W.K. Kellogg Foundation, Milbank Memorial Fund and the new Robert Wood Johnson Foundation.

Also often considered under the rubric of voluntary agencies are the many *associations* formed by professionals, agencies and institutions to further their mutual interests and professional goals. Examples are the American Medical Association, American Nurses' Association, American Hospital Association, American Public Health Association and the Association of American Medical Colleges.

Selected Readings

Voluntary Health and Welfare Agencies in the United States, Robert H. Hamlin. (New York: Schoolmaster's Press, 1961).

Voluntary Health Agencies, in *Public Health Administration and Practice*, Sixth Edition, John J. Hanlon (Saint Louis: The C.V. Masby Company, 1974).

Directories

Encyclopedia of Associations, Margaret Fisk, Ed. (Detroit: Gale Research Co.) An extensive listing of organizations, agencies and associations. Regularly updated.

The Foundation Directory, *Edition 5*, Marianna O. Lewis, Ed. (New York: The Foundation Center, 1975).

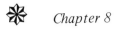 *Chapter 8*

Review and Control of Quality and Costs

1. QUALITY CONTROL

A common method of quality control in health as in other fields is the setting of basic minimal standards by public (governmental) and private (voluntary) agencies. The usual mechanisms are those of *licensure* (governmental), *accreditation*, and *certification* (voluntary).

Licensure

The states exercise the extensive licensing powers for health manpower and institutions. By appropriate legislation, the states may authorize persons who meet stated educational and, usually, examination criteria to engage in certain health occupations and professions. In addition to such *mandatory licensure*, some legislation merely authorizes use of a title to those meeting such criteria while not prohibiting others from engaging in the occupation (*voluntary licensure*). About 25 health occupations are licensed in some or all states,[1] either by mandatory (regulation of practice) or voluntary (protection of title) statutes. In addition to setting forth the general criteria, the legislation usually establishes boards of licensure or registration to implement the provisions, make rules and regulations

---

[1] Examples of personnel under mandatory licensure in all states are physicians, dentists, and pharmacists. Professional nurses have mandatory licensure in most states, but in several only the title (registered nurse) is protected.

and set procedures. Such boards are made up in large part of members of the profession being licensed.

The stimulus for licensure has traditionally come from professional groups and is often viewed as one manifestation of the process of "professionalization" of health occupations.

In addition to such regulation of manpower, the states also license hospitals and other health care institutions. In most cases this authority is vested by the legislature in the state health department. In some instances it is delegated to local city or county authorities.[2]

Accreditation

Accreditation is the process by which an institution or an educational program is determined to meet certain generally accepted standards set forth by an appropriate professional association. It is a voluntary process, and a hospital or program must apply to the accrediting agency for the necessary appraisal.

Examples of such accrediting bodies are the Joint Commission on Accreditation of Hospitals,[3] and the Liaison Committee on Medical Education, a joint committee of the American Medical Association and the Association of American Medical Colleges which accredits medical schools.

Certification

Certification (or registration)[4] is the process by which individual health personnel are affirmed to have attained a certain level of qualification, according to standards and criteria, such as education, experience and examination, set forth by their professional associations. These may be basic criteria for recognition of individuals as qualified to engage in the occupation, or may be criteria for recognition of advanced qualifications or specialization. An example of the former is the certified inhalation therapy technician certified by the American Association for Inhalation Therapy; examples of the latter are the medical specialties such as pediatrics and surgery which are certified by the specialty boards affiliated with the American Academy of Pediatrics and the American College of Surgeons.

[2] See also pages 40–49 on the regulation of health institutions.

[3] See page 34.

[4] The term "registration" may refer, depending on the context, to both licensure and certification. Board of licensure and certification boards are both often termed boards of registration or registries; also, the terms "license" and "certificate of registration" are often used interchangeably.

Medical Audit

In addition to these widely prevalent official and quasi-official mechanisms described above, the problem of evaluation and control of the quality of medical programs and institutions has been addressed in many other ways since the publication in 1910 of the most widely known single quality study, the Carnegie Commission's "Flexner Report" on medical education, resulting from a nationwide survey of medical schools.[5] Most of these efforts have been variations on the technique of *medical audit* which is broadly defined as the appraisal of quality by medical record review. This commonly has taken the form of analyses of individual cases, with judgments based on defined criteria for diagnosis and management, on expert opinion, or a combination of these.[6]

Professional Activity Study (PAS). The Professional Activity Study was begun in 1953 by the Southwestern Michigan Hospital Council and is now conducted by the Commission on Professional and Hospital Activities.[7] This program pioneered in the application of data processing techniques, first mechanical, then electronic, to the collection and analyses of medical record information on a large scale. Under this program, medical record personnel of participating hospitals abstract standard data from patient records at the time of hospital discharge. The data so obtained is then processed and reported to the hospital in the form of statistical summaries and case by case tabulations. Upwards of 1500 hospitals participate in the Professional Activity Study. The Medical Audit Program (MAP) is a related program whereby data are tabulated by clinical service, and in such a way as to facilitate review of patterns of professional practice.

2. COST CONTROL

Apart from the *claims review* systems long used by health insurance organizations, most of the formal activity related to the control of costs of health services has been by *utilization review*. This has

[5] Indeed, the origins of the Joint Commission on Accreditation of Hospitals lay in the proposals by the Clinical Congress of Surgeons, predecessor of the American College of Surgeons, for an analogous national survey of hospitals.

[6] This case analysis technique was first exemplified by the "end results" studies of Earnest A. Codman in 1912-1916.

[7] Under the sponsorship of the American College of Physicians, the American College of Surgeons, the American Hospital Association and the Southwestern Michigan Hospital Council.

generally been stimulated by concern regarding health insurance costs, and has been largely directed to institutional services, particularly hospital admissions.

Hospital Utilization Committees

It has been a long-time practice, especially during and after World War II, for the medical staffs of some hospitals with shortages of available beds and manpower, to establish committees to monitor admissions, including the setting of priorities. About 1960, however, the number of such committees began to increase, now largely under the pressures of health insurers and others, due to the rising costs of hospital care.[8]

Hospital Utilization Project of Pennsylvania (HUP)

This is a nonprofit organization sponsored by the Allegheny County Medical Society and the Hospital Council of Western Pennsylvania. It originated in 1963 as a pilot project set up to provide centralized assistance to a number of the area hospital review committees by providing computerized information on hospital discharges. It is an early example of such a regional, computerized process; about 100 Pennsylvania hospitals now use the expanded services of the Project.

Medicare Utilization Review

The Medicare legislation (Social Security Amendments of 1965) required that participating hospitals and extended care facilities have *utilization review plans.* This stipulation lead to the widespread formation of utilization review committees in these institutions as well as to considerable interest in the general problems of such review.

In recent years, as the costs of medical care have steadily risen, a wide variety of approaches to cost control have developed. Among these are the following:

[8] The most widely noted early example of such influences was the 1958 order of the Pennsylvania insurance commissioner to three Pennsylvania Blue Cross plans (which had requested rate increases) that steps must be taken to control costs. This led to the establishment of utilization committees in many Pennsylvania hospitals.

Certified Hospital Admission Program (CHAP)

This program was established in 1969 by the Sacramento California Foundation for Medical Care in cooperation with California-Western States Life Insurance Company. It provides review and certification (for payment) of hospital admissions; the process includes advance review of elective admissions and concurrent monitoring of length of stay.[9] (PAS data for area hospitals was initially used to develop length of stay criteria for the program.) Similar techniques for survey of admissions in advance or early in their course and for monitoring length of stay have become features of a number of other programs.[10]

"Certificate of Need" Statutes

Another recently developed mechanism of cost control is the "certificate of need" legislation which has been enacted by many states. These statutes are directed particularly at control of health facilities construction. Typically, facility construction must be approved by a designated state agency (usually the state health department, often with concurrence of the local [areawide] comprehensive health planning agency. Evidence that the proposed new or expanded facility is needed by the community must be presented. (See also page 48).

Prospective Reimbursement

Prospective reimbursement is a general term for mechanisms of payment for health care services at a rate determined in advance, as opposed to the traditional method of *retrospective reimbursement* for costs incurred. A number of states have established public *rate setting* bodies for this purpose. Systems have also been established by many Blue Cross plans.

3. COMBINED APPROACHES

There has been a general trend toward the integration of techniques for the systematic review of both utilization and quality. (Among

[9] Local (hospital) and regional (area) review committees use varying combinations of concurrent review (such as extended duration of stay) and retrospective review of hospital and nursing home admissions. The CHAP program adds the addition dimensions of prior review and certification for payment.

[10] For example, the Hospital Admission and Surveillance Program (HASP) of the Illinois Foundation for Medical Care, established in 1970, which monitors Illinois Medicaid admissions

many examples has been the use of PAS data by utilization review committees.) Important examples of programs and terminology include the following:

Peer Review

This term is often used for the general process of medical review of utilization and quality, when this is carried out directly or under the supervision of physicians; it often carries the implication that these will be practicing physicians.

Foundations for Medical Care

These are independent corporations sponsored by state or county medical societies which provide one or more services related to third-party payments to participating physicians. Declared common goals are the peer review of costs and quality of care in a fee-for-service context.

All foundations perform some type of review and monitoring of services and fees. Such activities range from review of claims referred by third-party payers (Medicaid programs, Blue Cross, Blue Shield and commercial insurance carriers) to the development of norms for medical procedures, hospitalizations, and length of stay for selected diagnoses. Some foundations sponsor prepaid health insurance plans, principally for employee groups, for which they provide complete claims processing including review and monitoring.

Most of the development of such foundations has taken place since 1965, and much of this since 1970, although the original organization, the San Joaquin Foundation for Medical Care, was established by the San Joaquin Medical Society in 1954. (This is the prototype for the foundations which sponsor complete prepaid health insurance plans.)

The *American Association of Foundations for Medical Care* gathers and distributes information about these organizations.

Quality Assurance Program (QAP)

This is a program sponsored by the American Hospital Association to expand and strengthen the activities of hospital-based utilization review and medical audit committees.

Performance Evaluation Procedure (PEP)

A Performance and Evaluation Procedure for Auditing and Improving Patient Care is an evaluation program developed by the Joint Commission on Accreditation of Hospitals. It has been designed as a methodology to facilitate hospitals' meeting the Commission's newly revised accreditation standards.

Experimental Medical Review Organizations (EMCRO)

This term is applied to a number of Foundations for Medical Care and other medical society-sponsored medical review organizations which participated, beginning in 1971, in a program sponsored and funded by the National Center for Health Services Research and Development, to develop models for the systematic review of physician services acceptable to professionals, the government and the public. The EMCRO program was developed in anticipation of the PSRO provisions of the 1972 Social Security Amendments. (See below)

Professional Standards Review Organizations (PSRO)

The establishment of these organizations was mandated by the Social Security Amendments of 1972 (Medicare-Medicaid amendments). They are associations of physicians organized to review professional and institutional services provided under the Medicare and Medicaid programs. The stated purpose of these organizations is the monitoring and control of both costs and quality.

Two hundred and three PSRO areas have been designated, for most of which Professional Standards Review Organizations have been established or planned. These have in general been sponsored by state and county medical societies, often through Foundations for Medical Care. (See above)

Selected Readings

1. *State Licensing of Health Occupations*, U.S. Department of Health, Education and Welfare, National Center for Health Statistics, 1967.

2. *Evaluation of the Medical Audit*, Paul A. Lembcke, Journal of the American Medical Association, 199:111, 1967.

3. *Evaluating the Quality of Medical Care*, Avedis Donabedian, Milbank Fund Quarterly, XLIV:166, 1966.

4. *The Utilization Committee*, Vergil N. Slee, in *The Medical Staff in the Modern Hospital*, by C.W. Eisele, Mc-Graw-Hill Book Company, New York, N.Y., 1967.

5. *Foundations for Medical Care*, Richard H. Egdahl, New England Journal of Medicine 288:491, 1973.

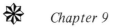 *Chapter 9*

The Pharmaceutical Industry
The Medical Supply and
Equipment Industry

1. PHARMACEUTICALS (DRUGS)

A basic distinction is made between:

Prescription drugs (also called *ethical drugs*) which are sold only to a person with a physician's prescription. Advertising for such drugs is directed only to physicians. Because these manufacturers follow this self-imposed ban on advertising these drugs to the public, these are sometimes called *ethical drugs* and their manufacturers the *ethical drug industry*.

Non-prescription drugs (*proprietary drugs, over-the-counter drugs, OTC's*) which are sold to the public without prescription and advertising is directed at the public audience (e.g. aspirin).

There are about 800 pharmaceutical manufacturers (drug companies) in the U.S. which make prescription drugs. (They may also make non-prescription drugs). Of these, about 135 of the largest, representing about 95% of all drug sales, belong to and are represented by the Pharmaceutical Manufacturers Association (PMA). The largest of these companies (based on dollar sales volume) are listed alphabetically in Table 9-1. Table 9-2 shows the application of the drug manufacturer's revenue dollar.

Table 9-1.   Total Sales, Major Drug Companies, 1972* ($ millions)

	Sales
Abbott Laboratories	521.8
American Home Products	1,578.0
Baxter Laboratories	278.8
Bristol Meyers	1,201.2
Johnson & Johnson	1,317.7
Eli Lilly & Company	819.7
Merck & Company	958.3
Miles Laboratories	319.0
Morton-Norwich	367.8
PEPI Inc.	203.7
Pfizer, Inc.	1,093.4
Richardson-Merrell	446.5
Schering-Plough	504.2
G.D. Searle & Company	271.9
Smith, Kline & French	402.3
Squibb Corporation	925.9
Sterling Drug	720.8
Upjohn Company	511.3
Warner Lambert	1,487.5

*Source: M. Silverman and P.R. Lee. Pills, Profits and Politics, (Berkeley: University of California Press), 1974, pp. 329–330.

List of Companies with sales over $200 millions in 1972. Note that some of these companies sell cosmetics and other non-drug products, and these sales dollars are included here. There are other very large companies which, among many products, sell some drugs. These companies are publicly owned. (Their stock shares are bought and sold in Stock Exchanges.)

Regulation: The Food and Drug Administration (FDA)

The Pure Food and Drug Act of 1906 specified that certain drugs are to be sold by prescription only and that the federal goverment is to insure that drug packages accurately state the names and quantities of the active ingredients. Before this time any drug including narcotics could be sold "over the counter" to the public. Impetus for this law came from the American Medical Association and the Muckrakers.

In 1927 the Food, Drug and Insecticide Administration was formed in the Department of Agriculture from the Bureau of Chemistry, which policed drugs prior to this time. In 1938, as a result of 100 deaths from a toxic sulfanilamide preparation, the Food, Drug and Cosmetic Act was passed which required that all new drug applicators (NDA) be submitted to the government prior to marketing to make sure that adequate toxicity studies had been made (Section 505).

Table 9-2. Where the Drug Manufacturer's Sales Dollar Goes

31.2	Cost of Goods Sold
2.5	Quality Control
15.5	Administration
0.7	Medical School Aid
20.0	Promotion (Advertising)
9.0	Research
12.0	Taxes
9.1	Profits

Source: *The Drug Makers and Drug Distributors.* (Washington: U.S. Government Printing Office, 1968), p. 13.

Required information for an NDA includes a full report on investigations in animals and humans to show that the drug is safe for use, a full statement of the composition of the drug, the method of its manufacture, and samples of labelling.

From 1938 to 1965 more than 14,000 NDAs were received. Special regulations were developed for investigational drugs to be used by experts. This law led to the problem of defining what is a new drug.

In 1953 the FDA became part of HEW.

In 1962, the Kefauver-Harris Drug Amendments were passed as a result of the Kefauver Senate Hearings on drug prices and the Thalidomide tragedy.

This required annual registration and inspection at least every two years of drug manufacturing establishments by the FDA. The FDA is empowered to regulate advertising, and to make a ruling that an NDA is sufficiently *safe* and *effective* before going on the market. The result is that the drug firm must undertake a substantial research and development effort to prepare an NDA.

Biologics

Biologics (biological products, biologicals) are any virus, therapeutic serum, toxin, anti-toxin, or analogous product applicable to the prevention of disease.[1] Biologics, including vaccines and blood plasma products, are regulated by the Bureau of Biologics, a division

[1] They differ from drugs in that biologics are usually derived from living microorganisms and cannot be synthesized or readily standardized by chemical or physical means. They tend to be chemically less stable than drugs, their safety cannot be as easily assured and they are never as chemically pure as drugs.

of the Food and Drug Administration (FDA), which in turn is part of HEW.

A key regulation in this area is the *Virus-Toxin Law of 1902* (*Biologics Control Act*) which was passed as a result of the deaths of a number of children from tetanus, effected by a contaminated diphtheria anti-toxin.

Licenses are granted for the manufacture and sale of biologics and annual inspection by the Division of Biologics Standards is required.

Naming Drugs

Drugs are known by three names:

1. The *chemical name* using the terminology that defines its chemical structure (e.g., 2 methyl-2 propyl-1, 3 propanediol dicarbamate).
2. The *generic name*: The established or official name for the drug (e.g., meprobamate).
3. The *brand name* (*proprietary drug name*): The registered trademark of a product given to it by its manufacturer (e.g., Miltown or Equanil).

Generic equivalents are similar drugs. There are three types of equivalency.

chemical equivalency. Drugs containing the same amount and type of active chemical equivalent.

biological equivalency. The chemical equivalents have the same *bioavailability* that is the same absorption rates, blood levels, and excretion rates.

clinical equivalency. The chemical equivalents have the same therapeutic effect on control of the disease or symptom.

A drug can be *an entity*: a simple chemical substance or biological product or a *combination*. It can be marketed in different dosage forms (e.g., tablets, syrups, solutions, etc.).

New drugs are patentable. A *patent* is a legal monopoly granted by the federal government for a period of 17 years from the time it is issued. A patent can cover new chemical entities, and new ways of making them, but not drug dosage forms. A company with a patented drug may license other companies to make and sell this drug in exchange for payment (royalties).

The patent is designed as a method for encouraging research and new ideas by allowing the inventor to "capture" the profits from his invention.

Antisubstitution Laws. About twenty years ago, nearly all states passed laws that forbid the pharmacist to substitute a chemical equivalent for the prescribed brand name drug. Recently, some of these state laws have been repealed. (Michigan)

The Structure of the Prescription Industry

The central importance of research for new drugs results in large research expenditures. The information and research necessary to process an NDA through the FDA is large and costly. Approval by the FDA and obtaining a patent and a trademark are the start of a marketing campaign which includes advertising to physicians in various forms and visits to doctors by *drug detail men*, who inform him of the use of this new product.

If there is no patent, other companies may make and sell the drug either under their own brand name or under the generic name. Drugs for sale by generic names are often sold at a substantially lower price. The critics of the industry argue that the difference results in vast monopoly profits from brand name drugs. The defenders of the industry argue that behind the brand name stands the reputation of the company for high quality performance and the price differential reflects quality differences. Usually only large drug firms can undertake this research and marketing process to develop new drugs. Promotional efforts are aimed almost entirely at physicians, who are legally the only ones allowed to write prescriptions.

Outside the hospital, prescriptions are filled only by registered pharmacists working in pharmacies licensed by the state. Pharmacies are either individually or chain owned (e.g., Rexall, Walgreens) and usually run for a profit. They also may provide a wide range of other products for sale which are not related to health. Pharmacists give some advice to patients concerning illness and remedies, particularly in the area of non-prescription preparations.

In 1970, of 2 billion prescriptions dispensed to patients, 46% were handled by about 50,000 independent community pharmacists (See Table 9-3); 39% by hospital pharmacies; 7% by chain pharmacies (usually 4 or more outlets centrally owned and operated). The re-

Table 9-3.   Pharmacies in the United States

	1973*	
Community Pharmacies	50,602	
Independent		39,998
Chain**		10,604
Hospital Pharmacies	5,174	

*National Association of Boards of Pharmacy *Licensure Statistics and Census of Pharmacy* Chicago, 1973

**Four or more pharmacies under the same ownership or management.

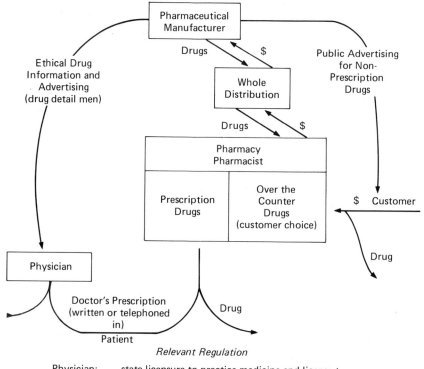

Diagram 9-1. Simplified Schematic Diagram of the Relationships between Pharmaceutical Manufacturers, Physicians, Pharmacists, and the Public

maining 8% by 1,500 pharmacies in department stores, supermarkets, etc., by mail order pharmacies, by doctors in their offices, and such.

Diagram 9-1 summarizes the key links between physician, pharmacist, and manufacturer.

References

L. Earle Arnow. *Health in a Bottle*. (Philadelphia: J.B. Lippincott Co., 1970).

Prescription Drug Industry Fact Book. Pharmaceutical Manufacturers Association. (Yearly).

Milton Silverman and Philip R. Lee. *Pills, Profits and Politics*. (Berkeley: University of California Press, 1974). This is the best source. The authors work hard to present both sides of the major issues, which is a rarity in the literature on the drug industry.

2. THE MEDICAL SUPPLY AND EQUIPMENT INDUSTRY

This includes manufacturers and distributors of radiographic and x-ray equipment, surgical and medical instruments and apparatus, and surgical appliances and supplies.

These include suture needles, orthopedic instruments, syringes and needles, anesthetic apparatus, hospital furniture, sterilizers, surgical dressings, adhesives, gauze and cotton, safety devices, hearing aids, artificial limbs, x-ray equipment, EEG's, EKG's, and such.

These manufacturing companies are independent, for-profit corporations. A sampling of larger American companies include:

American Hospital Supply	Englehard
American Optical	General Signal
American Sterilizer	Gulton
Beckman	International Rectifier
Becton-Dickinson	Profex-ray
Cenco	Telex
Cutter Labs	Textron

There are also large companies which produce many other types of products like:

Johnson & Johnson
Honeywell

Westinghouse
Bell & Howell
General Electric

Excluded from this industry are the whole range of companies that make everything from paper clips to computers, which are used in hospitals and health-related organizations.

Reference

R.D. Peterson, C.R. MacPhee, *Economic Organization in Medical Equipment and Supply*. (Lexington, Massachusetts: Lexington Books, 1973).

Appendices

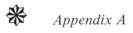 *Appendix A*

Alphabet Soup*

A	AABB	American Association of Blood Banks
	AAMC	Association of American Medical Colleges/ Association of American Medical Clinics
	AB	Aid to the Blind
	ACS	American College of Surgeons
	ADA	American Dental Association/American Dietetic Association
	AFDC	Aid to Families with Dependent Children
	AHA	American Hospital Association
	ALOS	Average Length of Stay
	AMA	American Medical Association
	AMHT	Automated Multi-Phasic Health Testing
	ANA	American Nurses' Association
	AOA	American Osteopathic Association
	APHA	American Public Health Association
	APTD	Aid to the Permanently and Totally Disabled
	ASCP	American Society of Clinical Pathologists
	AUPHA	Association of University Programs in Health Administration
B	BC	Blue Cross (Sometimes BX)
	BS	Blue Shield
C	CAP	Community Action Program

*This list contains abbreviations noted in the text.

	CARF	Commission on Accreditation of Rehabilitation Facilities
	CCU	Coronary Care Unit
	CDC	Center for Disease Control
	CHAMPUS	Civilian Health and Medical Program of the Uniformed Services
	CHAP	Certified Hospital Admission Program
	CHP	Comprehensive Health Planning
	CONUS	Continental United States (military hospitals)
	CPC	Clinico-Pathological Conference
	CT (ASCP)	Registered Cytotechnologist
	C&Y	Children and Youth Project
D	DAT	Dental Aptitude Test
	DAU	Dental Auxiliary Utilization
	DDS	Doctor of Dental Surgery
	DMD	Doctor of Dental Medicine
	DO	Doctor of Osteopathy
	DOD	Department of Defense
	DSC	Doctor of Surgical Chiropody
	DVM	Doctor of Veterinary Medicine
E	ECF	Extended Care Facility
	ECFMG	Educational Council for Foreign Medical Graduates
	EDDA	Expended Duty Dental Assistant
	EEG	Electroencephalograph
	EKG (ECG)	Electrocardiograph
	EMCRO	Experimental Medical Review Organization
	EPA	Environmental Protection Agency
	EPSDT	Early and Periodic Screening, Diagnosis and Treatment
	ER	Emergency Room
	EW	Emergency Ward
F	FDA	Food and Drug Administration
	FECA	Federal Employees Compensation Act
	FLEX	Federation Licensing Examination
	FMC	Foundation for Medical Care
	FMG	Foreign Medical Graduate
G	GHI	Group Health Insurance Plan
	GP	General Practitioner

H	HASP	Hospital Admission and Surveillance Program
	HEW	Department of Health, Education and Welfare
	HIAA	Health Insurance Association of America
	HIP	Health Insurance Plan of Greater New York
	HMO	Health Maintenance Organization
	HRA	Health Resources Administration
	HR 1	Social Security Amendments of 1972
	HSA	Health Services Administration
	HSA	Health Services Area; Health Systems Agency
	HSMHA	Health Services and Mental Health Administration
	HT (ASCP)	Histologic Technician
	HUD	Department of Housing and Urban Development
	HUP	Hospital Utilization Project of Pennsylvania
I	ICF	Intermediate Care Facility
	ICU	Intensive Care Unit
	IV	Intravenous
J	JCAH	Joint Commission on Accreditation of Hospitals
L	LPN	Licensed Practical Nurse
	LVN	Licensed Vocational Nurse
M	MA	Medical Assistance
	MCAT	Medical College Admission Test
	MCH	Maternal and Child Health
	MD	Doctor of Medicine
	MEDLARS	Medical Literature and Analysis Retrieval System
	MIC	Maternal and Infant Care Project
	MPH	Master of Public Health
	MSW	Master of Social Work
	MT	Medical Technologist
N	NASW	National Association of Social Workers
	NDA	New Drug Application
	NIH	National Institutes of Health

	NIMH	National Institute of Mental Health
	NIOSH	National Institute of Occupational Safety and Health
	NLN	National League for Nursing
	NMA	National Medical Association
O	OAA	Old Age Assistance
	OASDI	Old Age, Survivors and Disability Insurance (Social Security)
	OCD	Office of Child Development
	OD	Doctor of Optometry
	OEO	Office of Economic Opportunity
	OMB	Office of Management and Budget
	OPD	Outpatient Department
	OR	Operating Room
	OSHA	Occupational Safety and Health Administration
	OT	Occupational Therapist
	OTC	Over the Counter Drugs
P	PAS	Professional Activity Study
	PGP	Prepaid Group Practice
	PHS	Public Health Service (Also USPHS)
	PMA	Pharmaceutical Manufacturers' Association
	Pod. D.	Doctor of Podiatry
	PPC	Progressive Patient Care
	PR	Public Relations
	PSRO	Professional Standards Review Organization
	PT	Physical Therapist
Q	QAP	Quality Assurance Program
R	RMP	Regional Medical Program
	RN	Registered Nurse
	RPh	Registered Pharmacist
	RRL	Registered Record Librarian
S	SNF	Skilled Nursing Facility
	SRS	Social and Rehabilitation Service
	SSA	Social Security Administration
	SSI	Supplemental Security Income
T	TEAM	Training in Expanded Auxiliary Management

U	UR	Utilization Review
	USPHS	United States Public Health Service
V	VA	Veterans Administration
	VISTA	Volunteers in Service to America
	VMD	Doctor of Veterinary Medicine
	VNA	Visiting Nurse Association

Appendix B

Chronological List of Laws[1]

1902   Biologics Control Act

1906   Pure Food and Drug Act PL 59-384

1908   Federal Employees Compensation Act PL 60-176

1917   Vocational Education Act PL 64-347

1920   Vocational Rehabilitation Act PL 66-236

1921   Maternity and Infancy Act PL 67-97

1935   *Social Security Act PL 74-271

1943   Vocational Rehabilitation Amendments of 1943 PL 78-113
        Emergency Maternal and Infant Care Act PL 78-156

1944   *Public Health Service Act PL 78-410

1946   *National Mental Health Act PL 79-487
        *Hospital Survey and Construction Act PL 79-725
        *Vocational Education Act of 1946 PL 79-586

1949   *Hospital Survey and Construction Amendments of 1949
        PL 81-380

1954   *Medical Facilities Survey and Construction Act of 1954
        PL 83-482
        *Dependents Medical Care Act PL 24-569

[1] Major laws described or referred to in this book.
*Official short title.

1956   *Health Research Facilities Act of 1956 PL 84-835
*Health Amendments Act of 1956 PL 84-911
*National Health Survey Act PL 84-652

1958   Grants-in-Aid to Schools of Public Health PL 85-544

1959   *Federal Employees Health Benefits Act of 1959 PL 86-352

1960   *Social Security Amendments of 1960 PL 86-778
Graduate Training in Public Health PL 86-720

1961   *Community Health Services and Facilities Act of 1961 PL 87-395

1962   Health Services for Agricultural Migratory Workers PL 87-692

1963   *Health Professions Educational Assistance Act of 1963 PL 88-129
*Maternal and Child Health and Mental Retardation Planning Amendments of 1963 PL 88-156
*Mental Retardation Facilities and Community Mental Health Centers Construction Act of 1963 PL 88-164

1964   *Hospital and Medical Facilities Amendments of 1964 PL 88-443
*Economic Opportunity Act of 1964 PL 88-452
*Graduate Public Health Training Amendments of 1964 PL 88-497
*Nurse Training Act PL 88-581

1965   *Appalachian Redevelopment Act of 1965 PL 89-4
*Social Security Amendments of 1965 PL 89-97
*Mental Retardation Facilities and Community Mental Health Centers Construction Act Amendments of 1965 PL 89-105
*Heart Disease, Cancer and Stroke Amendments of 1965 PL 89-239
*Health Professions Educational Assistance Amendments of 1965 PL 89-290

1966   *Comprehensive Health Planning and Public Health Service Amendments of 1966 PL 89-749
*Allied Health Professions Personnel Training Act of 1966 PL 89-751

1967   *Mental Health Amendments of 1967 PL 90-31
*Mental Retardation Amendments of 1967 PL 90-170

*Partnership for Health Amendments PL 90-174
*Social Security Amendments of 1967 PL 90-248

1968   *Health Manpower Act of 1968 PL 90-490
        Public Health Service Amendments of 1968 PL 90-574

1969   *Federal Coal Mine Health and Safety Act of 1969 PL 91-173

1970   *Community Mental Health Centers Amendments of 1970 PL 91-211
        *Medical Facilities Construction and Modernization Amendments of 1970 PL 91-296
        *Communicable Disease Control Amendments of 1970 PL 91-464
        *Comprehensive Drug Abuse Prevention and Control Act of 1970 PL 91-513
        Public Health Service Amendments PL 91-515
        *Health Training Improvement Act of 1970 PL 91-519
        *Occupational Safety and Health Act of 1970 PL 91-596
        *Family Planning Services and Population Research Act of 1970 PL 91-572
        *Comprehensive Alcohol Abuse and Alcoholism Prevention, Treatment, and RehabilitationAct of 1970 PL 91-616
        *Emergency Health Personnel Act of 1970 PL 91-623
        *Lead-Based Paint Poisoning Prevention Act PL 91-695

1971   *Nurse Training Act of 1971 PL 92-158
        *Comprehensive Health Manpower Training Act of 1971 PL 92-157
        *National Cancer Act of 1971 PL 92-218
        Social Security Amendments PL 92-223

1972   *National Sickle Cell Anemia Control Act PL 92-294
        *Communicable Disease Control Amendments of 1972 PL 92-449
        *Social Security Amendments of 1972 PL 92-603
        *National Cooley's Anemia Control Act PL 92-714
        *Uniformed Services Health Professions Revitalization Act of 1972 PL 92-426
        *State and Local Fiscal Assistance Act of 1972 PL 92-512

1973   *Health Programs Extension Act of 1973 PL 43-45
        *Emergency Medical Services Systems Act PL 93-154
        *Health Maintenance Organization Act of 1973 PL 93-222

1974   *Sudden Infant Death Syndrome Act of 1974 PL 93-270
*Impoundment Control Act of 1974 PL 93-344 (Title X)
*Rehabilitation Act Amendments of 1974 PL 93-516
*National Health Planning and Resources Development Act of 1974 PL 93-641
*Headstart, Economic Opportunity and Community Partnership Act of 1974 PL 93-644
*Social Security Amendments of 1974 PL 93-647

1975   Public Health Service Amendments PL 94-63
*Developmentally Disabled Assistance and Bill of Rights Act PL 94-103

Appendix C

Summary of the Social Security Act (1935)

Title I   *Grants to the States for Old Age Assistance*

Provided grants to the states for financial assistance to needy aged.

Title II   *Federal Old Age Benefits*

Set up the federal "Social Security" program of old age benefits based on wages earned before age 65.[1]

Title III   *Grants to the States for Unemployment Compensation Administration*

Provided federal payment for the administrative expenses of state programs for unemployment compensation.

Title IV   *Grants to the States for Aid to Dependent Children*

Provided for grants to the states for financial aid for needy dependent children.[2]

---

[1] There were many exclusions in the original Act, including domestic and agricultural labor, employees of governmental and non-profit agencies, and the self-employed. Coverage since has been gradually extended and at present includes more than 90 percent of working people. (Railway workers are similarly covered under the Railroad Retirement Act; federal employees also have a separate program.)

[2] Children under age 16 deprived of parental support through death, absence or incapacity of a parent, and living with relatives. Payments are now authorized for children up to age 21 providing they are in school.

Title V   *Grants to the States for Maternal and Child Welfare*

Provided grants to the states for maternal and child health and child welfare services, and services to crippled children. Administration of the program was assigned to the Children's Bureau.[3] (Also extended vocational rehabilitation programs previously authorized under other legislation.)

Title VI   *Public Health Work*

Provided grants to the states for state and local public health services and additional funds for programs of the Public Health Service.

Title VII   *Social Security Board*

Established the Social Security Board to administer the programs authorized under the Act (with the exception of those in Titles V and VI), and to study and make recommendations regarding economic security and social insurance.

Title VIII   *Taxes with Respect to Employment*

Levied a payroll tax on employees eligible for the federal old age benefits program, and a tax in equal amount on their employers.

Title IX   *Tax on Employers of Eight or More*

Levied an additional tax on employers which could be credited against contributions to state unemployment funds. Its purpose was to encourage the establishment of such funds by the states.

Title X   *Grants to the States for Aid to the Blind*

Provided grants to the states for financial assistance to needy blind persons.

Title XI   *General Provisions*

Contained general definitions and administrative regulations.

---

[3] This Title in effect re-established and expanded the program of assistance for maternal and child health programs previously authorized under the federal Maternity and Infancy Act (1921–29) which was the first federal grant-in-aid program for direct health services.

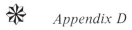 *Appendix D*

Social Security Amendments of 1965: Medicare*

Title XVIII, Health Insurance for the Aged

Part A: Hospital Insurance Benefits. This insurance program provides basic protection against the costs of hospital and related post-hospital services. Benefits consist of entitlement to have payment made for:

- *Inpatient hospital* services up to 90 days during any spell of illness and psychiatric inpatient services up to 190 days lifetime.
- Post-hospital *extended care* services up to 100 days during any spell of illness.
- Post-hospital *home health* services up to 100 visits in a one-year period.
- Hospital outpatient diagnostic services.

The amount payable for these services (except home health) is subject to deductible and coinsurance payments by the beneficiary as follows:

- *Inpatient*: $40 deductible until January 1, 1969, thereafter to be increased according to the increase in average per diem rates for in-hospital services;[1] coinsurance, equal to one-fourth the deductible, for each day after the sixtieth hospital day.

*Summary

[1] The deductible was considered to represent roughly the cost of the first hospital day.

- *Extended care*: no deductible; coinsurance, equal to one-eighth the inpatient hospital deductible, for each day after the twentieth day.
- *Home health services*: no deductible or coinsurance.
- *Outpatient*: for services provided in a 20-day period by one hospital, deductible is equal to one-half the inpatient deductible; coinsurance is equal to 20 percent of the remaining amount payable.

The *conditions for payment to providers* of service include:

- Written request by beneficiary (except where found impracticable by the Secretary).
- *Certification* by a physician of the necessity for the services, and periodic recertification where applicable, beginning no later than the twentieth day.
- For psychiatric hospital services, certification that such treatment can reasonably be expected to *improve the condition* for which treatment is necessary.
- For tuberculosis hospital services, certification that treatment can reasonably be expected to *improve the condition* or render it non-communicable.
- For post-hospital extended care services, certification of the need for *skilled nursing care* for condition for which the preceding inpatient services were received.
- For post-hospital home health services, certification that services are required because the individual is confined to his home and needs *skilled nursing care*, or physical or speech therapy for conditions for which he was receiving inpatient hospital services.

The amount paid to any provider of services must be the *reasonable cost* of such services.

Payment may be made for emergency services provided by a non-participating hospital including, under limited conditions, hospitals outside the United States.

Groups of associations of providers of services may elect to have payments made through a public or private agency or organization.[2] The Secretary is authorized to make agreements with such designated organizations by which they will determine the payments to be made for services and will make such payments. These agencies may be required to:

- Provide consultation to providers for their establishment of necessary fiscal records and the meeting of other qualifications.

[2] These non-federal agencies which deal directly with the providers of services are known as *fiscal intermediaries.*

- Serve as a center for communication of information between the Secretary and the providers.
- Make necessary audits of records of providers.

The nomination of an agency or organization, however, is not binding on individual members of the nominating association or group.

A *Federal Hospital Insurance Trust Fund* is established for payments under Part A. The trust fund is to be financed by an earnings tax paid by employees, employers and the self-employed.

Part B: Supplementary Medical Insurance Benefits. This is a voluntary insurance program financed from premium payments by enrollees and contributions from federal funds. Benefits consist of entitlement to have payment made for:

- Home health services up to 100 visits in a year.
- Medical and other health services:
  a. *physicians'* services
  b. *services and supplies* incident to a physician's professional services
  c. *diagnostic X-ray*, laboratory, and other tests
  d. *radio-therapy*
  e. *surgical dressings*, splints, casts
  f. *rental of durable medical equipment* used in the home
  g. *ambulance service* (with limitations)
  h. *prosthetic devices* (except dental) and *braces*

Independent laboratories providing services under this program must be approved by the Secretary.

Payments for *physicians' services* are to be 80 percent of *reasonable charges*, and may be made to the beneficiary or on his behalf. (An organization providing services on a prepayment basis may be paid 80 percent of reasonable costs.)

Payments for other medical and health services are to be 80 percent of *reasonable costs*.

Medical and other health services under this part are subject to a $50 deductible in each calendar year. (Expenses incurred for hospital outpatient diagnostic services under Part A may be counted toward the deductible.)

With regard to out of hospital *psychiatric services*, there shall be considered as incurred expense in any year, no more than $250 after the deductible.

The *conditions for payment to providers* of services include:

- Written *request by beneficiary*, unless impracticable.
- In the case of *home health* services, *certification by a physician* that the individual is confined to his home and needs skilled nursing care or physical or speech therapy and that services are furnished while the individual is *under the care of a physician.*
- In the case of other medical or health services, certification by a physician, that these were *medically required.*

Provision is made for general and individual *enrollment periods.*

The *initial monthly premium is set at $3.* Beginning in 1968, the monthly premium shall be determined every two years on the basis of the benefit and administrative costs of the program.

For persons receiving monthly Social Security benefits, premiums will be deducted from these payments.

A *Federal Supplementary Insurance Trust Fund* is established for payments under Part B.

The Surgeon General is authorized to enter into *contracts with (health insurance) carriers* for administration of these benefits. The carriers will:

- Determine rates and amounts of payments required, disburse and account for funds, and make necessary audits of records of providers of services.
- Assist in development of procedures relating to utilization practices and determine compliance with requirements for utilization review.
- Serve as a channel for communication of information relating to the administration of this program.
- Assure that payments are made for reasonable costs, and for charges which are reasonable and not higher than the charges applicable for comparable services to the policyholders and subscribers of the carrier. Payments for charges may be made on the basis of a receipted bill or on the basis of an *assignment.* In the latter case the reasonable charge will be the full charge for the services.

In determining the reasonable charge for services there shall be taken into consideration the *customary charges* for similar services generally made by physicians or other persons furnishing such services, as well as the *prevailing* charges in the locality.

The Surgeon General, at the request of a state, will enter into an agreement whereby eligible individuals in the federally aided *public assistance categories* will be enrolled in Part B with the monthly premium to be paid by the state.

A government contribution will be made from the Treasury *equal to the aggregate premiums* payable under this part.[3]

Part C: Miscellaneous Provisions. Definitions[4] (for purposes of Title XVIII) include:

- Spell of Illness—a period beginning with the first day on which an individual is furnished inpatient hospital services or extended care services and ending with the close of the first period of 60 consecutive days thereafter on each of which he is neither an inpatient of a hospital or an extended care facility.
- Inpatient Hospital Service
  a. Bed and board.
  b. Such nursing services, use of hospital facilities, medical social services, and such drugs, biological supplies, appliances, and equipment, for use in the hospital, as are ordinarily furnished to in-patients by a hospital.

  Excluded are *physicians'* services (except interns and residents under a training program) and the services of *private duty nurses.*
- Hospital—an institution which:
  a. Is primarily engaged in providing by or under the supervision of physicians, to in-patients, services for diagnosis, treatment, care, or rehabilitation.
  b. Maintains clinical records on all patients.
  c. Has bylaws in effect with respect to its staff of physicians.
  d. Has a requirement that every patient must be under the care of a physician.
  e. Provides *24-hour nursing service* rendered or supervised by a registered professional nurse.
  f. Has in effect a hospital *utilization review plan.*
  g. If in any state whose laws provide for licensing of hospitals, is so licensed or meets the standards for licensure.
  h. Meets such other requirements as the Secretary finds necessary in the interest of the health and safety of hospitalized individuals except that such requirements may not be higher than the comparable requirements of the Joint Commission on Accreditation of Hospitals.

[3] i.e., half the costs of Part B will be paid from general revenues.

[4] Abbreviated.

- Extended Care Facility[5] —an institution (or distinct part of an institution) which has in effect a *transfer agreement* with one or more participating hospitals and which:
  a. Is primarily engaged in providing to inpatients *skilled nursing care* or *rehabilitation* services.
  b. Has policies which are developed with the advice of a group of professional personnel, and has a physician, a registered professional nurse or a medical staff responsible for the execution of such policies.
  c. Requires that every patient be under the supervision of a physician and provides for having a physician available in case of emergency.
  d. Maintains clinical records on all patients.
  e. Provides *24-hour nursing service* sufficient to meet nursing needs in accordance with the policies developed and has *at least one registered nurse employed full time.*
  f. Provides appropriate methods and procedures for the dispensing and administering of drugs and biologicals.
  g. Has a *utilization review plan.*
  h. If in any state with laws providing for licensing of such institutions, is so *licensed* or meets the licensure standards.
  i. Meets such other conditions relating to the health and safety of its patients as the Secretary may find necessary.
- Utilization Review—a utilization review plan of a hospital or extended care facility is considered sufficient if it is applicable to services to individuals entitled to insurance benefits under this title. It is to provide:
  a. For a review, on a sample or other basis, of admissions, *duration of stay* and professional services with respect to *medical necessity* and to promote the most efficient use of facilities and services.
  b. For review to be made by a staff committee of *two or more physicians*, with or without other professional personnel or a similar group established by the local medical society and some or all of the hospitals and extended care facilities in the locality.
  c. For review of cases of *extended duration.*
  d. For prompt notification to the institution, the individual, and his physician of any finding (made after opportunity for consultation with such physician) that further stay in the institution is not medically necessary.
- Home Health Agency—an agency or organization which:

---

[5] This term has since been superseded by the term *Skilled Nursing Facility.*

a. Is primarily engaged in providing skilled nursing services and other therapeutic services.
b. *Has policies established by a group of professional personnel* including one or more physicians and one or more registered professional nurses, and provides for supervision of such services by a physician or a registered professional nurse.
c. Maintains clinical records on all patients.
d. If in any state providing for the licensing of organizations of this nature, is so *licensed* or meets the licensure standards.
e. Meets *such other conditions of participation* as the Secretary may find necessary in the interest of individuals furnished services.

- Home Health Services—the following items and services furnished to an individual under the care of a physician by a home health agency on a visiting basis in an individual's home:
  a. Nursing care provided by or under the supervision of a registered professional nurse.
  b. *Physical, occupational*, or *speech* therapy.
  c. Medical *social services.*
  d. *Home health aid* services.
  e. Medical *supplies* and use of medical *appliances.*
  f. Any of the foregoing provided on an outpatient basis at a hospital, extended care facility, or rehabilitation center which involves the use of equipment which cannot be made readily available in the home.
- Post-Hospital Extended Care Services—extended care service furnished an individual after transfer from a hospital in which he was an inpatient for not less than *3 consecutive days*; admission to the extended care facility to be not more than *14 days* after discharge from such hospital.
- Post-Hospital Home Health Services—home health services furnished an individual within one year after his most recent discharge from a hospital of which he was an inpatient for not less than *3 consecutive days*, or from an extended care facility (in which he was an inpatient under Part A). In either case, the plan for home health services is to be established *within 14 days* after such discharge.
- Physician—a licensed doctor of medicine, osteopathy, or dentistry.
- Provider of Services—a hospital, extended care facility, or home health agency.

Payment is to be made for the reasonable cost of *semi-private* accommodations: two-bed, three-bed, or four-bed. Payment may exceed semi-private cost only if more expensive accommodations are required for medical reasons. If accommodations furnished are less expensive than semi-private, payment will be minus the difference.

Excluded from coverage are (among others):

- Services which are not provided within the United States (except emergency services).
- Personal comfort items.
- Routine physical *checkups*; *eyeglasses* or related eye examinations; *hearing aids* or related examinations; *immunizations*.
- *Orthopedic* shoes or other supportive devices for the feet.
- *Custodial care*.
- *Cosmetic surgery except* as required for repair of accidential injury or improvement of functioning of a malformed body member.
- Care, treatment, filling, removal, or replacement of teeth.
- Services provided under a workmen's compensation law.

In developing *conditions of participation for providers of services* the Secretary shall consult with the Health Insurance Benefits Advisory Council, appropriate state agencies, recognized national listing or accrediting bodies and may consult with appropriate local agencies.

The Secretary shall make an agreement with any state willing and able to do so whereby an appropriate state or local agency may determine whether an institution is a hospital or extended care facility, or an agency is a home health agency (as these terms are defined) or whether a laboratory meets the stated requirements. The Secretary may also agree to utilize the services of such agencies to:

> Provide consultation to institutions or agencies to assist them to establish and maintain fiscal records or otherwise to qualify as providers of services, including the establishment of utilization review procedures.

The requirements for a participating hospital shall be deemed to have been met if an institution is accredited as a hospital by the *Joint Commission on Accreditation of Hospitals* (provided that utilization review procedures are also established).[6]

A *Health Insurance Benefits Advisory Council* of 16 members is established to advise the Secretary on general policy in the administration of this Title and in the formulation of regulations. Members to include persons in fields related to hospital, medical and other health activities and at least one person representing the general public.

---

[6] Accreditation by the American Osteopathic Association or other national accreditation body may also be accepted.

A *National Medical Review Committee* of 9 members is established to include individuals who are representative of organizations and associations of professional personnel in the field of medicine, other individuals from medicine or related fields, and at least one member representative of the general public; a majority of the members to be physicians. The function of the Committee is to study the utilization of hospital and other medical care and services provided under this Title with a view to *recommending any changes* which may seem desirable *in the way in which such services are utilized* and in the *administration of the programs* established by this Title.

The Secretary shall *prescribe such regulations* as may be necessary to carry out the administration of this program.

Eligibility. Persons eligible are those who have attained the age of 65 and are entitled to monthly social security or railroad retirement benefits. Other persons are eligible under transitional provisions, provided they attain age 65 before 1968 and are resident citizens of the United States or have been permanent resident aliens for at least five years. Excluded are those eligible for the Federal Employee Health Benefits Program and those convicted of specific crimes against national security.

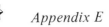 *Appendix E*

Social Security Amendments of 1965: Medicaid *

Title XIX, Grants to the States for Medical Assistance Programs

"For the purpose of enabling each state to furnish medical assistance on behalf of families with dependent children and of aged, blind, or permanently and totally disabled individuals whose income and resources are insufficient to meet the costs of necessary medical services . . ."

This Title establishes a single *new program of medical assistance* for persons receiving federally aided public assistance[1] and extends eligibility to comparable groups of *medically indigent persons*, i.e., needy families with dependent children, and blind, disabled or elderly persons who are not on welfare. All *needy children* (under 21) are also made eligible.

The federal share of the program's costs is 53–80 percent, according to a state's per capita income.

Participation in the new medical assistance program is optional for the states, who can elect to continue (until January 1970) under the old medical provisions of the public assistance titles. After January 1970 federal payments for medical care of the medically indigent aged (Kerr-Mills program) will be made only under the new program, which would now have to include the other groups as well. A state not

*Summary

[1] Persons eligible for Aid to Families with Dependent Children, Old Age Assistance, Aid to the Blind, and Aid to the Permanently and Totally Disabled.

starting the new program by January 1970 may no longer receive federal funds for medical care under the public assistance programs.

In states electing to implement the new program, all persons on public assistance (federally aided categories) are to be included. The same program of services is to be made available to all persons included in the program, except that states electing to include aged persons in mental and tuberculosis hospitals are not required to extend the same services to persons under 65.

As a minimum, a medical assistance program must include (at least some of each of) the following:

- Inpatient hospital services
- Outpatient hospital services
- Other laboratory and X-ray services
- Skilled nursing home services
- Physicians' services

Additional services which the States may make available are:

- Medical care furnished by licensed practitioners
- Home health care services
- Private duty nursing services
- Clinic services
- Dental services
- Physical therapy and related services
- Prescribed drugs, dentures, prosthetic devices, and eyeglasses
- Other diagnostic, screening, preventive, and rehabilitation services
- Inpatient hospital and skilled nursing home services for individuals 65 or over in tuberculosis or mental hospitals
- Any other medical care recognized under State Law.

The States are required to show progress toward broadening the scope of services available and liberalizing the (State's) eligibility requirements for medical assistance with a view toward furnishing, by July 1, 1975, *comprehensive services to substantially all individuals meeting the State's eligibility standards* with regard to income and resources.

No durational residence requirements may be imposed nor any lien against a recipient's property during his lifetime, or lifetime of spouse and surviving minor children. Financial responsibility of relatives other than for spouse or minor children may not be taken into account for purposes of determining eligibility.

Payment for inpatient hospital services is to be made on the basis of *reasonable cost.*

A single state agency is to be designated to administer the medical assistance program except that the determination of eligibility shall be made by the agency administering the program for *old age assistance* [in effect, the State's Department of Public Welfare].

Social Security Amendments of 1965: Maternal and Child Health*

Title V, Maternal and Child Health and Crippled Children's Services

- Increased grant funds are authorized for maternal and child health and crippled children's services.
- Grants are authorized for *training professional personnel* for care of crippled children, particularly children with multiple handicaps.
- Special Project Grants for Health of School and Pre-school Children.

Grants are authorized for "projects of a comprehensive nature for health care and services for *children and youth* of school age or for pre-school children" particularly in areas with concentrations of low income families.

Grants may be made to a state or local health agency, the agency administering the Title V programs, to any school of medicine (with appropriate participation by a school of dentistry) or to any affiliated teaching hospital.

Projects are to include at least such screening, diagnosis, preventive services, treatment, correction of defects, and aftercare, both medical and dental, as may be provided for in regulations of the Secretary.

Treatment, correction of defects, or aftercare provided under the project is to be available only to children *who would not otherwise*

*Summary

265

receive it because they are from low income families or for other reasons beyond their control.

- Payments for inpatient hospital services are to be made on the basis of *reasonable costs.*
- Increased grant funds are authorized for child welfare services.

Index

Tissue Committee (hospital medical
staff), 18
Title 18. (*See* Medicare.)
Title 19. (*See* Medicaid.)
TPR (temperature, pulse, and respiration), 19
training grants, 139-140, 173
Training in Expanded Auxiliary Management (TEAM), 76
Transportation, Department of, 7, 9
Treasury, Department of, 122, 124
triage, 217
tuberculosis, 10, 12, 13, 162, 165,
174, 203, 204, 205, 206, 212,
219

umbrella agencies, 206-207
unemployment compensation (insurance), 124, 160, 249
Uniformed Services Health Professions
Revitalization Act of 1972, 118
unit manager, 21, 23, 78
United Cerebral Palsy Association, 35
United States Code, 137, 200
United States Government (see Federal
government)
unmet need, 103
unwed mothers, homes for, facility
for, 2, 33
upper limit on coverage (insurance),
91
usual and customary fee, 89
utility regulation, 46, 48
utilization review, 223-224
hospital medical staff committee,
18, 224
Medicare, 152, 156, 224, 256

vendor payments, 102, 104, 110-113
venereal disease control, 124, 162,
165, 166, 174, 204, 206, 212
Veteran's Administration, (VA), 120-
121, 123
Department of Medicine and Surgery,
120
hospitals, 7-9, 46, 87, 110-113, 121
veterinary medicine, veterinarians, 52,
58, 60, 65, 85, 122, 177, 178,
191

Virus-Toxin Law of 1902, 232
vision care (see eye care), 183
Visiting Nurse Association (VNA),
Visiting Nurse Service, 3, 213-
214, 219
VISTA. *See* Volunteers in Service to
America, 119, 198, 199
vital statistics, 131, 162, 204
Vocational Education Act of 1917, 79
Vocational Education Act of 1946,
176
Vocational Rehabilitation Act amendments (1943), 125
Vocational Rehabilitation, Office of,
123, 125
vocational rehabilitation, 125, 126,
135, 199, 204
professions, 58, 60, 65
expenditures on, 111-113
voice (regulation), 40, 44, 46, 47
voluntary agencies, 219-220
voluntary hospitals, 6, 7, 11-12
voluntary staff, 211
Volunteers, hospital (see auxiliary),
21, 28, 31
Volunteers in Service to America
(VISTA), 119

waiting list (hospital), 15
waiver (insurance), 91
walk-in patient, 217
ward clerk, 23, 30, 65
ward patients, 13
Water, Public Water Systems, 192
Weed Lawrence L., M.D., 19
welfare, 124, 199
Welfare Administration, 126
work training and work study programs (Economic Opportunity
Act), 197
Workmen's Compensation, 98-99,
110-113

X-ray. *See* radiology, 4, 5, 31, 84, 183,
235

Youth development, office of, 128,
129